HAEMODIALYSIS

Other titles in the *New Clinical Applications* Series:

Dermatology (Series Editor Dr J. L. Verbov)
Dermatological Surgery
Superficial Fungal Infections
Talking Points in Dermatology – I
Treatment in Dermatology
Current Concepts in Contact Dermatitis
Talking Points in Dermatology – II
Tumours, Lymphomas and Selected Paraproteinaemias
Relationships in Dermatology

Cardiology (Series Editor Dr D. Longmore)
Cardiology Screening

Rheumatology (Series Editors Dr J. J. Calabro and
Dr W. Carson Dick)
Ankylosing Spondylitis
Infections and Arthritis

Nephrology (Series Editor Dr G. R. D. Catto)
Continuous Ambulatory Peritoneal Dialysis
Management of Renal Hypertension
Chronic Renal Failure
Calculus Disease
Pregnancy and Renal Disorders
Multisystem Diseases
Glomerulonephritis I
Glomerulonephritis II

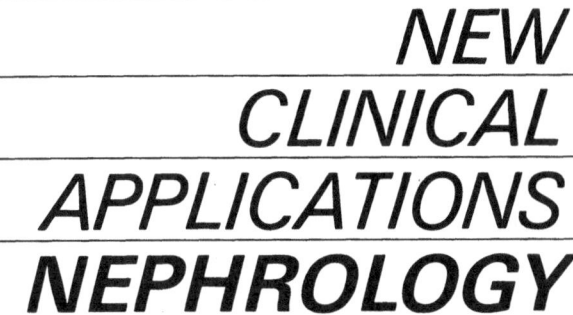

NEW
CLINICAL
APPLICATIONS
NEPHROLOGY

HAEMODIALYSIS

Editor

G. R. D. CATTO
MD, DSc, FRCP (Lond., Edin. and Glasg.)

Professor of Medicine
University of Aberdeen
UK

KLUWER ACADEMIC PUBLISHERS
DORDRECHT / BOSTON / LONDON

Distributors

for the United States and Canada: Kluwer Academic Publishers, PO Box 358, Accord Station, Hingham, MA 02018–0358, USA
for all other countries: Kluwer Academic Publishers Group, Distribution Center, PO Box 322, 3300 AH Dordrecht, The Netherlands

British Library Cataloguing in Publication Data

Haemodialysis.
  1. Man. Kidneys. Haemodialysis
  I. Catto, Graeme R.D. (Graeme Robertson
  Dawson). *1945–*   II. Series
  617′.461059

Library of Congress Cataloguing in Publication Data

Haemodialysis/editor, G.R.D. Catto.
     p.   cm.—(New clinical applications. Nephrology)
  Includes bibliographies and index.
  ISBN-13: 978-94-010-7058-4   e-ISBN-13: 978-94-009-1257-1
  DOI: 10.1007/978-94-009-1257-1

  1. Hemodialysis.   I. Catto, Graeme R.D.
  [DNLM: 1. Hemodialysis. WJ 378 H1335]
  RC901.7.H45H34 1988
  617′.461059—dc19
  DNLM/DLC
  for Library of Congress   88–37909
                        CIP

Copyright

Published in the United Kingdom by Kluwer Academic Publishers,
PO Box 55, Lancaster, UK.

Kluwer Academic Publishers BV incorporates the publishing programmes of D. Reidel, Martinus Nijhoff, Dr W. Junk and MTP Press.

CONTENTS

List of Authors   vi

Series Editor's Foreword   vii

About the Editor   viii

1. Acetate or bicarbonate for haemodialysis?   1
   N. T. Richards and A. J. Wing

2. Haemofiltration   33
   A. M. Martin and M. I. McHugh

3. Clinical haemoperfusion   61
   J. F. Winchester

4. Anticoagulation for haemodialysis   83
   I. S. Henderson

Index   106

LIST OF AUTHORS

I.S. Henderson
Renal Unit
Dundee Royal Infirmary
Dundee DD1 9ND
UK

A.M. Martin
Department of Renal Medicine
The Royal Infirmary
New Durham Road
Sunderland SR2 7JE
UK

M.I. McHugh
Department of Renal Medicine
The Royal Infirmary
New Durham Road
Sunderland SR2 7JE
UK

N.T. Richards
Renal Laboratory
St Thomas' Hospital
Lambeth Palace Road
London SE1 7EH
UK

J.F. Winchester
Division of Nephrology
Georgetown University Medical Cent
3800 Reservoir Road NW
Washington DC 20007
USA

A.J. Wing
Renal Laboratory
St Thomas' Hospital
Lambeth Palace Road
London SE1 7EH
UK

SERIES EDITOR'S FOREWORD

For more than a generation haemodialysis has been the principal method of treating patients with both acute and chronic renal failure. Initially, developments and improvements in the system were highly technical and relevant to only a relatively small number of specialists in nephrology. More recently, as advances in therapy have demonstrated the value of haemoperfusion for certain types of poisoning, the basic principles of haemodialysis have been perceived as important in many areas of clinical practice.

In this volume, the potential advantages of bicarbonate haemodialysis are objectively assessed, the technical and clinical aspects of both haemofiltration and haemoperfusion discussed and the continuing problems associated with such extracorporeal circuits analysed. All the chapters have been written by recognized experts in their field. The increasing availability of highly technical facilities for appropriately selected patients should ensure that the information contained in the book is relevant not only to nephrologists but to all practising clinicians.

ABOUT THE EDITOR

Professor Graeme R. D. Catto is Professor in Medicine and Therapeutics at the University of Aberdeen and Honorary Consultant Physician/Nephrologist to the Grampian Health Board. His current interest in transplant immunology was stimulated as a Harkness Fellow at Harvard Medical School and the Peter Bent Brighton Hospital, Boston, USA. He is a member of many medical societies including the Association of Physicians of Great Britain and Ireland, the Renal Association and the Transplantation Society. He has published widely on transplant and reproductive immunology, calcium metabolism and general nephrology.

1
ACETATE OR BICARBONATE FOR HAEMODIALYSIS?

N. T. RICHARDS AND A. J. WING

Thomas Graham, a Scotsman who lived from 1805–1869, demonstrated that vegetable parchment acts as a semipermeable membrane[1]. He coated parchment with albumin to close any defects then stretched it over a wooden or guttapercha hoop which he floated in a tank of water. Into the hoop he put a combination of crystalloid and colloid and demonstrated that only the crystalloid diffused through the parchment into the water. Graham coined the term dialysis for this phenomenon. He later repeated the experiment using urine and again showed that only the crystalloid matter passed into the water, and that when the water was evaporated to dryness it yielded a white crystalloid powder which was mainly urea. Graham was a chemist rather than a physician and as such did not apply dialysis to animals.

It was not until 1913 that Abel, Turner and Rowntree[2] from Baltimore described a method 'by which the blood of a living animal may be submitted to dialysis outside the body, and again returned to the natural circulation without any exposure to air, infection by microorganisms or any alteration which would necessarily be prejudicial to life'. Numerous investigators used the technique on animals but it was not until 1924 that George Haas[3] from Gieszen, Germany, performed the first human dialysis. The first patient to owe her life to dialysis was treated by Willem Kolff[4] using a rotating drum dialyser, constructed by himself and Hendrik Berk working in Kampen, Holland in 1945. The dialysis fluid used in the early attempts at dialysis was either saline or isotonic Ringer's solution. Kolff performed numerous studies on the formulation of dialysis fluid. Though he was hampered by the lack of modern analytical techniques he suggested the following composition (converted from mg%):

sodium	126.5 mmol/L
potassium	5.4 mmol/L
calcium	1.0 mmol/L
bicarbonate	23.9 mmol/L
chloride	109.0 mmol/L
dextrose	76 or 151 mmol/L

The major problem with formulation was the alkalinity caused by the bicarbonate which further affected the solubility of calcium and magnesium, leading to the precipitation of calcium and magnesium carbonate. Kolff attempted to resolve this problem by bubbling CO_2 into the dialysate, but this proved technically too difficult. He resolved the problem by not adding calcium to the tap water (1 mmol/L) and giving calcium gluconate intravenously at the end of dialysis[5]. The problem was solved by other workers in different ways. Murray[6] added sodium phosphate and sodium carbonate, which had also been tried by Kolff. Alwall[7] employed a closed container for both the dialyser and dialysis fluid and was thus able to bubble CO_2 into the fluid to reduce the pH. Skeggs and Leonards[8] used both CO_2 and phosphate. Eventually, the accepted method for the majority of early dialysis systems became to use bicarbonate as the base and to bubble either 5% or 10% CO_2 continuously through the dialysate to lower the pH. The problem with this system led to a search for an alternative source of base.

In the early 1960s the choice was between acetate and lactate. The initial step in acetate metabolism is conversion to acetyl CoA, which sits at the crossroads of many metabolic pathways (Figure 1.1). It is estimated that more than 90% will be metabolized via the Krebs cycle leading to the production of ATP and the regeneration of bicarbonate (Figure 1.2). The remaining 10% may be metabolized in either of two ways: acetyl CoA may be converted to malonyl CoA and used in fatty acid synthesis (Figure 1.3), or it may be converted to acetoacetyl CoA, which may be used in ketone body and cholesterol synthesis (Figure 1.4).

2

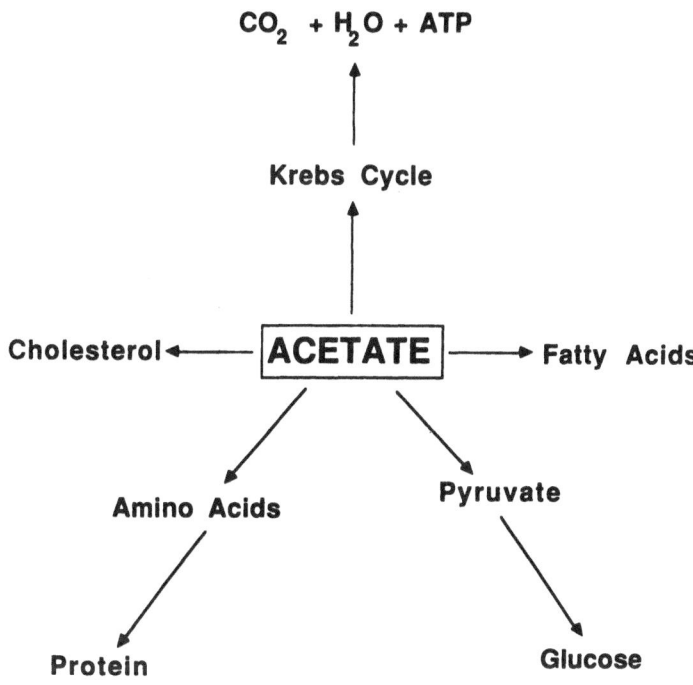

FIGURE 1.1   Acetate sits at the crossroads of many metabolic pathways

Mion, whilst working with Scribner[9] in Seattle, noted work by Lundquist[10] who estimated that, in normal subjects, the maximum rate of acetate utilization was 300 mmol/h, a value arrived at indirectly from alcohol loading. In 1964, they published a clinical trial describing the use of a dialysate in which all the bicarbonate had been replaced with acetate. Its use was studied in six patients with chronic renal failure. They found the dialysance of acetate (55–65 ml/min) to approximate to that of bicarbonate (55–70 ml/min) and that a dialysate concentration of 35–40 mmol/L was required to maintain a serum bicarbonate concentration of approximately 20 mmol/L. Their patients suffered no adverse effects when dialysed against acetate, even with dialysate acetate concentrations of up to 120 mmol/L.

Following this report, acetate was universally accepted as the standard dialysate buffer and has remained so for over 20 years. In 1982,

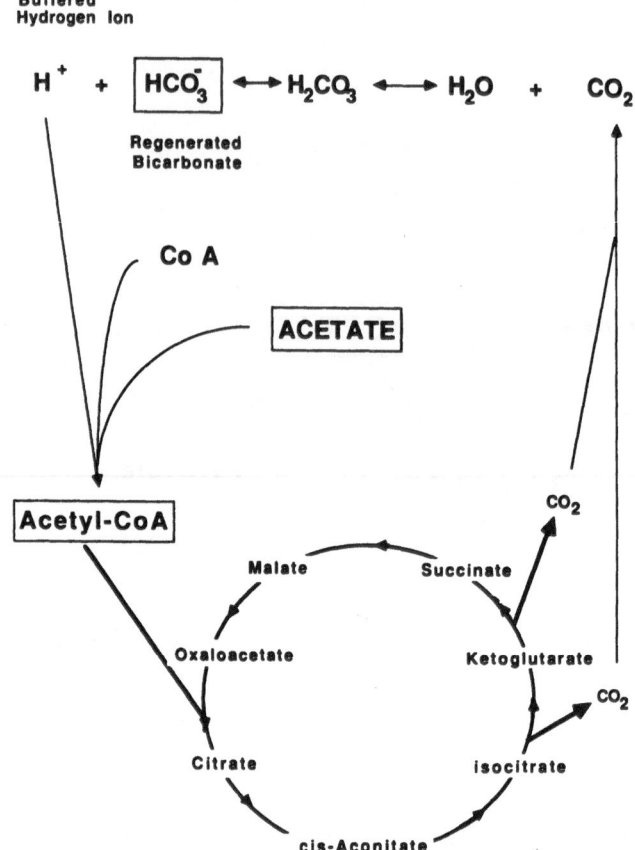

FIGURE 1.2   Regeneration of bicarbonate during the metabolism of acetate via the Krebs cycle

figures from the European Dialysis and Transplantation Association (EDTA) suggested that 94% of dialyses used acetate as the source of base. However, in the last decade, a number of reports have accumulated which suggest that its use contributes to dialysis morbidity. The technology allowing for on-line proportioning of bicarbonate dialysate is now available (Figure 1.5) and this, along with the advent of rapid high-efficiency dialysis, has led to an increase in the use of bicarbonate as the dialysate buffer. Figures from the EDTA for 1986 suggest that

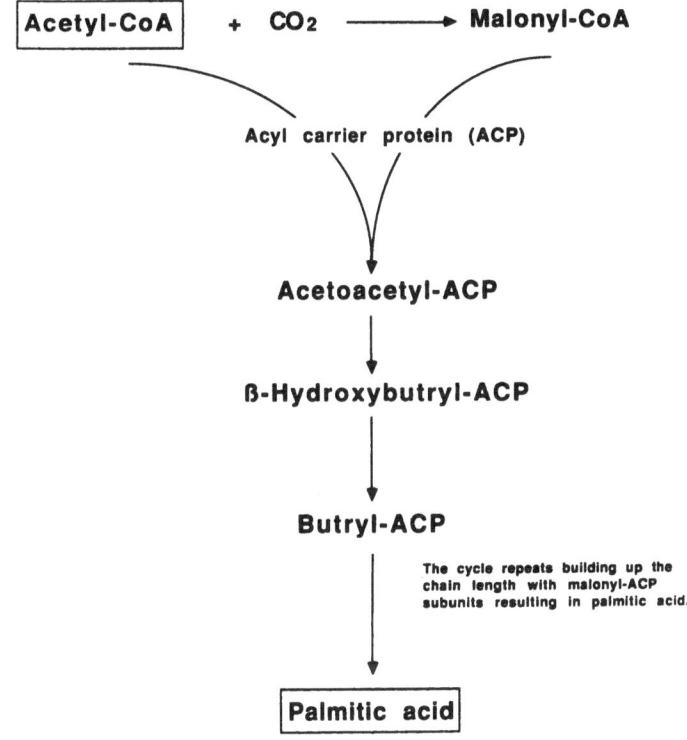

FIGURE 1.3   Fatty acid synthesis

the bicarbonate dialysate is used in 20% of dialyses.

DIALYSIS-RELATED SYMPTOMS. ACETATE INTOLERANCE?

The term 'acetate intolerance' was first coined by Novello et al.[11] in 1976. They described a study of nine nephrectomized patients (3 children and 6 adults) undergoing routine haemodialysis. Following the initiation of dialysis, six patients demonstrated a rapid rise in blood acetate concentrations to no more than 8.2 mmol/L. Three patients achieved levels exceeding 15 mmol/L. Two of these experienced persistent acidosis and episodes of hypotension with nausea, vomiting, headache and chills, though the symptoms were not necess-

5

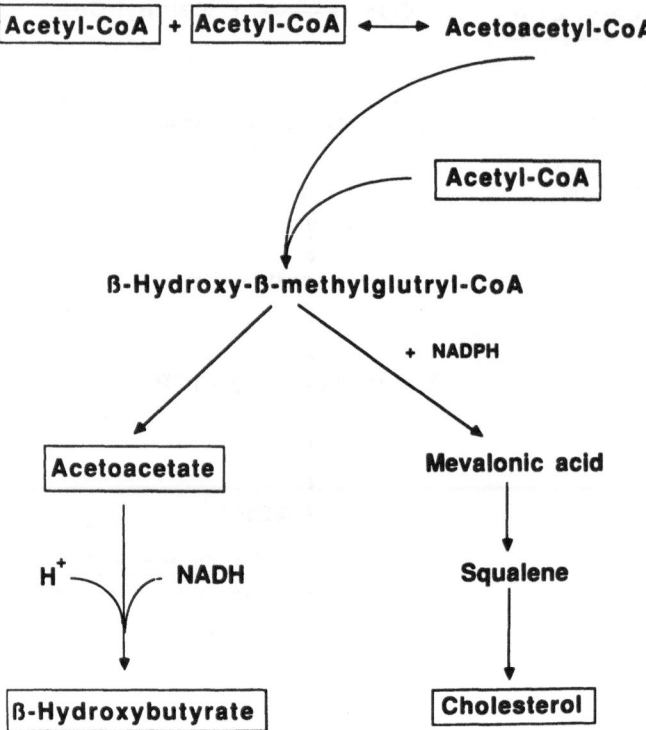

FIGURE 1.4   Ketone body and cholesterol synthesis

arily related to the high acetate levels. Graefe *et al.*[12] in 1978 studied six patients, selected because of symptoms during dialysis. During acetate dialysis with large dialysers, there was a marked fall in plasma bicarbonate and pCO_2 throughout the dialysis. Plasma bicarbonate increased rapidly to above normal levels at the end of the dialysis, with a return of pCO_2 to base-line values. During bicarbonate dialysis, these changes were largely eliminated. Using a double-blind protocol (neither the nursing staff, attending physicians or patients were aware of which dialysate was being used), symptoms occurred in 85% of acetate dialyses compared with 17% of bicarbonate dialyses. The use of bicarbonate in the dialysate permitted the tolerable rate of ultrafiltration to be increased by 67% more than that possible with acetate.

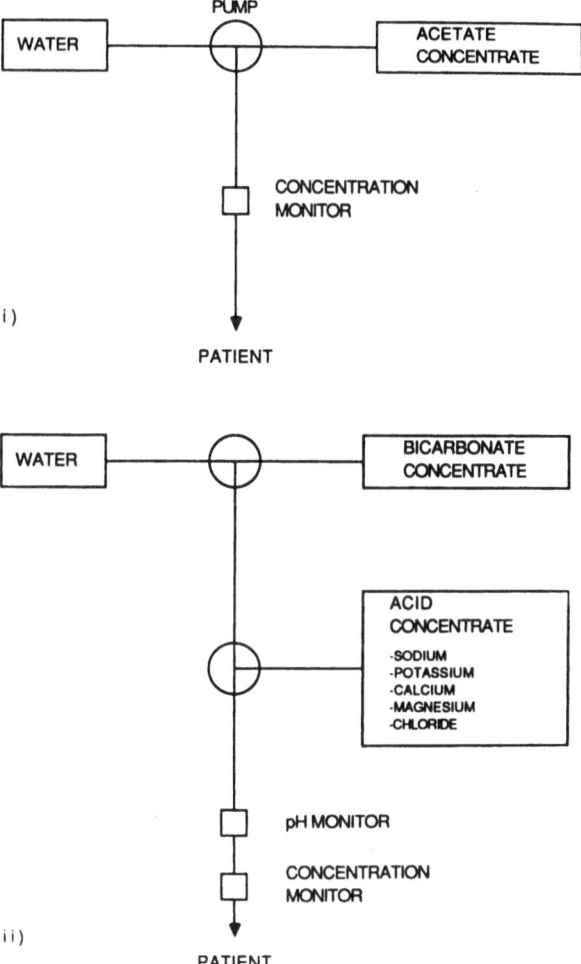

FIGURE 1.5   Schematic representation of the 'on line' production of acetate (i) and bicarbonate (ii) dialysates

The above two studies are largely responsible for the concept that intradialytic symptoms, such as nausea, vomiting, headache, hypotension and post-dialysis fatigue, are caused by 'acetate intolerance' and may be alleviated by the substitution of bicarbonate for acetate in the dialysate.

A large volume of work has since been published on the concept of

7

acetate intolerance with greatly conflicting results. The cause of this conflict is largely related to differences in experimental design. Many variables other than the dialysate buffer must be considered. Not least of these is the net mass transfer of acetate to the patient. This is dependent upon the duration of the dialysis, blood and dialysate flow rates, the dialyser surface area and permeability and the concentration of acetate used. Other factors affecting the interpretation of these studies include: the dialysate sodium concentration, the methods for measurement and interpretation of plasma acetate levels and the selection of patients.

Dialyser surface area

In the UK at present, standard dialysis employs the use of dialysers with a surface area in the range $0.8–1.2\,m^2$. The transfer of acetate to the patient during the same duration of dialysis will thus be much less than that seen by Graefe with the use of dialysers of $2.5\,m^2$. Studies conducted using dialysers in the range $0.8–1.5\,m^2$ to assess the benefit of bicarbonate over acetate, with respect to symptoms, give conflicting results. Patel et al.[13] described 12 stable chronic haemodialysis patients. Half dialysed with $1.0\,m^2$ and half with $1.4\,m^2$ dialysers, against a dialysate sodium of 130 mmol/L. They found no difference in symptoms, no accumulation of acetate, acetate uptake or bicarbonate loss. Bijaphala et al.[14] studied eight patients in a double-blind manner using $1.1\,m^2$ dialysers over ten months and found no benefit of bicarbonate over acetate in amelioration of symptoms. Hakim et al.[15] in 16 chronic haemodialysis patients studied over a three month period, showed no difference in symptoms between the use of acetate or bicarbonate dialysate. However, in a subgroup of elderly patients who experienced hypotension during acetate dialysis, the number of episodes were decreased by the use of bicarbonate dialysate. Velez et al.[16] in 1984 looked at the contribution of autonomic neuropathy to symptom production, but was only able to show a benefit of bicarbonate over acetate when dialysing against a low dialysate sodium. The only study to show a benefit of bicarbonate over acetate whilst using standard dialysers was that by Man et al.[17] in a study that was neither blind nor crossover. They studied 18 patients on bicarbonate dialysis and

8

15 on acetate dialysis over a 2-year period using 1 m^2 polyacrylonitrile dialysers. Significantly fewer episodes of hypotension, nausea, headache and muscle cramps occurred during bicarbonate dialysis.

Numerous studies have been performed using dialysers in the range 1.5–2.5 m^2. In these, a different picture emerges. Van Stone and Cook[18], with a double-blind study of nine randomly selected patients using 1.5 and 2.5 m^2 dialysers, used a state of well being index to show that patients felt better after bicarbonate dialysis than after acetate dialysis. Moderate to severe symptoms occurred 2.5 times more frequently during acetate than bicarbonate dialysis. Similar results have been obtained by Uldal et al.[19], Klopp et al.[20] and Pagel et al.[21]. Klopp used continuous EEG monitoring and showed that a normal alpha pattern was only found during bicarbonate dialysis, the tracing becoming markedly abnormal during acetate dialysis with development of a superimposed beta pattern concomitantly with symptoms and the onset of hypocapnia. Pagel measured choice reaction time (CRT) (the time in milliseconds taken to make a decision about the colour of a flashing panel) before and immediately after each dialysis. Reaction time was significantly greater during both acetate dialysis and dialysis against a combination dialysate containing acetate 38 mmol/L and bicarbonate 10 mmol/L. Increasing acetate levels were associated with increased deterioration in CRT scores. The findings of the studies outlined above are summarized in Table 1.1.

Dialysate sodium concentration

Alterations in the dialysate sodium concentration affect intradialytic symptoms[22–25] and must be considered when studying the effect of different dialysate buffers. Others have combined alteration of sodium concentration with change in dialysate buffer. Shimizu et al.[26], in 1983, studied 28 patients in a double-blind trial of high (142 mmol/L) against low (135 mmol/L) sodium, in combination with acetate or bicarbonate as buffer. They showed a beneficial effect of high sodium and bicarbonate dialysate, bicarbonate mitigating against fatigue and high sodium against cramps and headache. Velez et al.[16] 1984, in a double-blind study of 12 patients, 7 with autonomic neuropathy, showed that bicarbonate was only of benefit in the presence of low sodium

TABLE 1.1   Summary of studies comparing acetate with bicarbonate dialysate in relation to intradialytic symptoms

Authors	Number of patients	Study design	Dialyser size	Findings
Novello et al.[11]	9	NB CO	?	Persistent acidosis in 2 patients
Graefe et al.[12]	6 Symptomatic	DB CO	2.5 m²	Bicarbonate superior
Van Stone et al.[18]	9	DB CO	1.5 m² (5) 2.5 m² (4)	Bicarbonate superior
Uldall et al.[19]	16	DB CO	1.8 m²	Bicarbonate superior
Klopp et al.[20]	6 Symptomatic	NB CO	?	Bicarbonate superior
Pagel et al.[21]	21	NB CO	1.8 m²	Bicarbonate superior
Man et al.[17]	15 (acetate) 9 (bicarbonate)	NB NC	1.0 m²	Bicarbonate superior
Patel et al.[13]	12	NB CO	1.0 m² (6) 1.4 m²	No difference
Velez et al.[16]	13	DB CO	1.0 m²	No difference
Bijaphala et al.[14]	8	SB CO	1.1 m²	No difference
Hakim et al.[15]	16	DB CO	0.8 m²	No difference

(NB = not blind; DB = double blind; SB = single blind; CO = crossover; NC = not crossover)

(131 mmol/L) dialysate, having no advantage over acetate when the dialysate sodium was high (141 mmol/L). 1.0 m² dialysers were used. Bijaphala et al.[14] studied 8 patients with a single-blind technique using 1.1 m² dialysers. They showed that high sodium (139 mmol/L) was superior to low sodium (132 mmol/L) in terms of blood pressure control, fluid removal and symptoms during dialysis, but could find no benefit of bicarbonate over acetate. The findings of the studies outlined above are summarized in Table 1.2.

TABLE 1.2 Summary of studies comparing high and low sodium and acetate and bicarbonate dialysates in relation to intradialytic symptoms and incidence of hypotension

Author	Number of patients	Study design	Sodium (mmol/L) High	Low	Findings
Shimizu et al.[26]	28	DB CO	142	135	High Na superior to low bicarbonate prevents fatigue
Velex et al.[16]	12	DB CO	141	131	Bicarbonate superior to acetate with low sodium dialysate
Bijaphala et al.[14]	8	SB CO	139	132	No advantage of bicarbonate over acetate
Wehle et al.[39]	6	NB CO	145	133	Slight benefit of bicarbonate with low sodium dialysate
Henrich et al.[46]	10	DB CO	140	—	Reduced therapeutic intervention with bicarbonate
Hsu et al.[95]	6	DB CO	144	134	Bicarbonate superior with low sodium dialysate

(DB = double blind; SB = single blind; NB = not blind; CO = crossover)

Blood acetate concentrations

Acetate is difficult to measure[11,27]. Many of the studies which cite 'acetate intolerance' as a cause of symptoms during dialysis have not measured acetate levels[12,17,18,26]. Novello et al.[11] in 1977 were the first to describe rising acetate levels during dialysis.

Mansell *et al.*[28] developed a sensitive rapid direct gas chromatographic method for measurement of plasma acetate. Plasma acetate levels in normal subjects vary between 0.01 and 0.4 mmol/L. Mansell *et al.*[28] studied 20 adult and 4 paediatric patients undergoing dialysis for end-stage renal failure, as well as four patients with acute hepatorenal failure. In 75% of the adults and all of the children, arterial acetate levels stabilised after one hour of dialysis at 2.4 and 2.2 mmol/L respectively. 25% of the adults showed a progressive rise in acetate levels during dialysis to values greater than 5.3 mmol/L and, in one case, reached 15.5 mmol/L.

Acetate flux was measured during dialysis and shown to be the same in all patients. The incidence of hypotension, vomiting and malaise was no greater in those patients who developed high acetate levels. The 5 patients with combined renal and liver failure did not develop high acetate levels, despite glucose intolerance and circulatory failure. Rising acetate levels during dialysis have been described by others[12,19,21] but none have convincingly demonstrated a correlation between symptoms and high plasma acetate levels. There is no evidence that the 25% of people who are slow metabolizers of acetate are the same 25% who are likely to experience symptoms.

Weiner[29] in 1979 performed acetate kinetic modelling studies on normal subjects and on dialysis patients. In normal subjects, acetate obeys first order kinetics whilst acetate kinetics in dialysis patients was best fitted to a Michealis–Menton model (first order at concentrations less than 2 mmol/L, zero order at concentrations above 2 mmol/L). He showed that patients with a $V_{max} > 14$ mmol/L would show a rise in bicarbonate levels during acetate dialysis, whilst patients with a $V_{max} < 7$ mmol/L would have a fall in bicarbonate levels during dialysis, and thus be more likely to develop worsening acidosis during acetate dialysis.

Recently, Mansell *et al.*[30] have measured acetate levels in 12 patients undergoing bicarbonate dialysis. Commercial bicarbonate concentrate contains 4–10 mmol/L acetate. In 10 of this group, no change was found, but, in 2 patients, the acetate levels increased to 1.5–2.0 mmol/L. Both these patients had been shown to have normal acetate levels during acetate dialysis.

Working on the hypothesis that large infusions of acetate may lead to high acetaldehyde concentrations, Cairns *et al.*[31] have measured arterial acetaldehyde levels during acetate and bicarbonate dialysis in 15 patients. They showed that, in 5 of the subjects, the acetaldehyde levels increased steadily after two to three hours of dialysis and continued to increase 30 min post-dialysis. No hypotensive episodes occurred in these patients. Blood acetate and acetaldehyde concentrations directly correlated.

In summary (Tables 1.1 and 1.2), in our opinion, in the presence of a dialyser surface area less than $1.5 m^2$ and a dialysate sodium concentration greater than 137 mmol/L bicarbonate has not been clearly shown to be a superior buffer to acetate. Anecdotal observations suggest that a number of patients experience less symptoms when using bicarbonate dialysate, but the double-blind studies have shown how misleading such observations may be. In the presence of large surface area dialysers or a low dialysate sodium concentration, the use of bicarbonate as the buffer may result in fewer and less severe episodes of hypotension and less symptoms, in particular nausea and fatigue. Furthermore, ultrafiltration appears to be better tolerated during bicarbonate dialysis.

CARDIOVASCULAR STABILITY

Myocardial performance may be abnormal in uraemic patients for several reasons: (a) anaemia, (b) hypertension, (c) coronary artery disease, (d) autonomic dysfunction, (e) pericardial disease and (f) the toxic effects of uraemia itself.

The question of whether acetate (a) has a direct cardiodepressant action or (b) causes cardiovascular instability indirectly by peripheral vasodilatation and reflex tachycardia during dialysis, is extremely controversial. The studies performed to answer these questions are beset with the same problems as discussed above, namely patient selection, failure to use a randomized, double-blind protocol, differences in mass transfer of acetate and failure to control for osmolality changes during dialysis with an appropriate dialysate sodium concentration (see Table 1.3).

Early experiments by Kirkendol et al.[32] in dogs and then Aizawa et al.[33] in man suggested that acetate has a direct cardiodepressant action which is responsible for cardiovascular instability seen during acetate

TABLE 1.3 Summary of studies on the effect of acetate on myocardial contractility during haemodialysis in patients with acute and chronic renal failure and during acetate infusion

Author	Method	Preload	Afterload	Heart rate	Contractility
Aizawa et al.[33]	PET/ET	?	Reduced	Unchanged	Depressed
Iseki et al.[36]	Dye dilution	?	Reduced	Unchanged	Enhanced
Nixon et al.[40]	Echo	Unchanged	Unchanged	Unchanged	Enhanced
Chen et al.[35]	Echo	Reduced	Reduced	Unchanged	Enhanced
Shick et al.[42]	Echo	?	Reduced	Increased	Enhanced
Nitenberg et al.[38]	Thermo-dilution	Unchanged	Unchanged	Paced	Enhanced
Vincent et al.[48]	Thermo-dilution	Reduced	Reduced	Increased	Depressed
Huyghebaert et al.[49]	Thermo-dilution	Unchanged	Reduced	Unchanged	Depressed

(PET = pre-ejection period; ET = left ventricular ejection time)

dialysis. Originally, Kirkendol injected massive bolus doses of acetate but later infused it slowly[34] to show that acetate caused a dose-dependent increase in cardiac output, stroke volume and stroke work, with a marked reduction in systemic vascular resistance. Aizawa assessed cardiac function by the use of the ratio of the pre-ejection period to left ventricular ejection time, calculated from simultaneous phono- and electrocardiography, a technique since invalidated[35]. Iseki et al.[36] studied 6 patients and observed a fall in mean arterial pressure accompanied by an increase in cardiac index during acetate, but not bicarbonate, dialysis. Canella et al.[37], in a study of 11 patients, corroborated the finding of a fall in mean arterial pressure with acetate, but not bicarbonate, dialysis.

Nitenberg et al.[38] performed sodium acetate infusions in non-uraemic subjects undergoing cardiac catheterization for ischaemic heart disease. Changes in heart rate were eliminated by atrial pacing. Plasma acetate levels were elevated to a mean of 3.1 mmol/L (com-

14

patible with those seen during acetate dialysis[28]). They demonstrated an increase in cardiac index, ejection fraction, maximum velocity of shortening, end systolic stress–end systolic volume ratio and total body oxygen consumption. Direct injection into the left coronary artery caused no change in heart rate, LV end systolic and diastolic pressures, or positive dP/dt_{max}. Thus, the enhancement of myocardial contractility seen during the acetate infusion did not result from a direct effect of acetate on the myocardium.

Wehle et al.[39] attempted to dissociate the haemodynamic effects of ultrafiltration and diffusion dialysis. Six patients were studied during isolated ultrafiltration and then during ultrafiltration with dialysis. The independent variables included acetate, bicarbonate, high sodium (145 mmol/L) and low sodium (133 mmol/L) dialysates. Systolic blood pressure and mean arterial pressure, which were stable during isolated ultrafiltration, fell slightly when the high dialysate sodium was used and much further when the dialysate sodium concentration was low. These changes were related to changes in plasma osmolality. Acetate had no effect on blood pressure at high sodium concentrations, but a slight (not significant) effect when used in the low-sodium dialysate. Nixon et al.[40] performed a similar study employing echocardiography to assess left ventricular function. They studied patients during isolated ultrafiltration, routine dialysis and isovolumetric dialysis, in a group of patients not receiving any cardiac or antihypertensive drugs. Ventricular performance was plotted over several cardiac-filling volumes. It was concluded that ultrafiltration alone produced a pure Frank Starling effect (a decrease in end diastolic volume, a leftward shift in the ventricular function curve), while haemodialysis, with or without volume loss, produced an upward shift in the ventricular function curve. Recent studies[41–45] have been performed on more homogeneous groups of patients, some in a double-blind crossover fashion[46] and most utilizing mean velocity of circumferential fibre shortening (Vcf) as a measure of cardiac performance. These have demonstrated a similar positive inotropic effect, with a comparable improvement in cardiac function with both acetate and bicarbonate. The study of Ruder et al.[45] was only able to show an improvement in Vcf during acetate dialysis in patients with abnormally low Vcf prior to dialysis.

Apart from the work of Nitenberg et al.[38], the above data relate to patients with chronic renal failure who have been receiving regular

15

haemodialysis. There have been four studies of patients with acute renal failure. The first, by Borges et al.[47], studied 30 patients over 120 dialyses with a double-blind, crossover protocol. Four patients had diabetes and two liver failure. None required artificial ventilation or received vasoactive drugs. Intracardiac monitoring was not used. There were no differences in symptoms, mean blood pressure, number of hypotensive episodes or rates of ultrafiltration between acetate and bicarbonate dialysis. pCO_2 and pH were lower in the acetate group at the second hour of dialysis.

The studies of Vincent et al.[48], Huyghebaert et al.[49], and Leunissen et al.[50] all contradict the findings of Borges. Intracardiac monitoring was used in all cases. All three studies included ventilated patients, although no patients received vasoactive drugs. Vincent showed that blood pressure and cardiac output fell to a similar degree with both dialysates, but, during acetate dialysis, there was a greater increase in heart rate and a significantly lower left ventricular stroke work index during and up to 30 min after acetate dialysis. Greater volumes of intravenous saline were needed to maintain blood pressure during acetate dialysis. Serum bicarbonate and pH decreased during acetate dialysis. Huyghebaert studied septic patients with acute renal failure. Although heart rate and systemic vascular resistance did not change significantly during use of either buffer, decreases in cardiac output and mean arterial pressure were more pronounced during acetate dialysis. Leunissen documented significant falls in mean arterial pressure and left ventricular stroke work index during acetate dialysis, which did not occur during bicarbonate dialysis. pO_2 and pCO_2 fell during acetate dialysis. The difference between the results of Borges et al.[47] and those of Vincent et al.[48], Huyghebaert et al.[49] and Leunissen et al.[50] may be explained by the lack of severely ill patients in Borges' study, as judged by the fact that none required ventilatory or inotropic support.

In summary (Table 1.3), the use of bicarbonate as the dialysate buffer does not appear to confer greater cardiovascular stability during routine dialysis of patients with chronic renal failure and normal left ventricular function. Bicarbonate has been shown to be superior to acetate in the presence of poor left ventricular function, a low dialysate sodium concentration and, most importantly, in the critically ill patient with acute renal failure.

PULMONARY PERFORMANCE

Johnson *et al.*[51] first described hypoxaemia during haemodialysis in 1970. This observation has been corroborated and appears to occur with both acetate[19,52] and bicarbonate[47,52] dialysates. The reduction in the arterial oxygen tension (PaO_2) is usually only between 10–15 mmHg, but its clinical importance is suggested by the fact that a number of dialysis-related symptoms may be alleviated by the administration of oxygen[53]. This drop in PaO_2 has been attributed to a variety of events, including:

(1) The formulation of microemboli, resulting in interference with intrapulmonary gas exchange[54];

(2) Dialyser membrane-induced complement activation, leading to pulmonary leucostasis[55];

(3) Changes in oxygen transport and ventilation due to production of a metabolic alkalosis (the Bohr effect);

(4) Reflex hypoventilation secondary to loss of CO_2 via the dialyser[56];

(5) Increased consumption of O_2 and decreased production of CO_2 during the metabolism of acetate[57];

Craddock *et al.*[55,58] noted that profound transient neutropenia occurred in patients within the first 30 min of dialysis, the total neutrophil count dropping to about 20% of predialysis values. This was associated with a decrease in the transfer factor, an increase in the alveolar–arterial oxygen gradient and a fall in pO_2. The fall in neutrophil count is at its greatest at 30 min and recovers within one hour, whilst hypoxaemia lasts for the whole dialysis[59,60]. When cellophane membranes are used for isolated ultrafiltration, neutropenia occurs in the absence of hypoxia[59,61]. Complement activation may be prevented by the use of polyacrylonitryl or polysulphone membranes, but hypoxaemia still occurs during dialysis with these membranes, albeit to a lesser extent[60,62].

Increasing the pH of the blood increases the affinity of haemoglobin for oxygen (the Bohr effect) which decreases oxygen tissue delivery. The relative alkalosis produced also leads to a fall in alveolar ventilation by a direct action on the respiratory centre. In practice, these mechanisms are unlikely to be important. Haemodialysis hypoxaemia has been shown to occur in the absence of changes in pH[63]; acetate dialysis results in increasing acidosis rather than alkalosis in the early stages of dialysis[12] and hypoxaemia is improved by the use of bicarbonate dialysate, despite the presence of alkalosis[64].

The respiratory centre is extremely sensitive to changes in pCO_2. During acetate dialysis, CO_2 is excreted down a concentration gradient through the dialyser resulting in a fall in the pCO_2 and thus a fall in alveolar ventilation, resulting in hypoxia. This is supported by several studies in which CO_2 loss through the dialyser has been estimated[56,62,65], and by the observation that, when CO_2 is bubbled into the dialysate, or bicarbonate is exchanged for acetate, hypoxia was lessened[56]. Unfortunately, when these studies are examined in greater depth, it may be seen that the calculated losses of CO_2 through the dialyser have been exaggerated by the inclusion of both bicarbonate and CO_2.

Oh *et al.*[57,66] suggest that acetate metabolism via the Krebs cycle leads to an increase in oxygen consumption. Acetate enters the Krebs cycle by conversion via acetyl CoA to citric acid. In the process, 1 mmol of CO_2 is consumed and 1 mmol of HCO_3^- is generated (Figure 1.2). Citric acid is then further metabolized, leading to the production of two mmol CO_2 and the consumption of two mmol O_2. Thus, for each mmol CO_2 produced, 2 mmol O_2 are consumed; hence acetate metabolism leads to a decline in the respiratory quotient (RQ).

$$RQ = CO_2 \text{ production}/O_2 \text{ consumption}$$

From the alveolar gas equation:

$$PAO_2 = FiO_2 - PaCO_2/RQ$$

where PAO_2 is the partial pressure of oxygen in the alveolus and FiO_2 the inspired oxygen tension. It can be seen that a fall in RQ results in a fall in PAO_2 and hence PaO_2.

In summary, the aetiology of dialysis-induced hypoxaemia is multifactorial and the main contributing factor has yet to be elucidated. The use of bicarbonate dialysate leads to less hypoxaemia than the use of acetate dialysate, as does the use of more biocompatible dialyser membranes. The effects of the two are additive. However, even the use of bicarbonate dialysate and a more biocompatible membrane will not completely abolish the hypoxia of haemodialysis.

18

ACID–BASE BALANCE AND INTERMEDIARY METABOLISM

Replenishment of bicarbonate buffer stores depleted by interdialytic acid generation is an important goal of dialysis therapy. It has been suggested that the use of bicarbonate, rather than acetate, dialysate leads to better correction of the metabolic acidosis[67],[68]. This may be beneficial in the prevention of dialysis-related morbidity, poor growth in children[69] and the progression of metabolic bone disease. However, several groups have failed to show an improvement in correction of metabolic acidosis with the use of bicarbonate dialysate[14,30,70].

Buffer repletion relies on generation of bicarbonate from the metabolism of acetate (Figure 1.2). The involvement of the Krebs cycle is reflected by increasing concentrations of citrate seen during acetate dialysis[71]. The initial step in acetate metabolism is the formation of acetyl CoA, utilizing 1.0 mmol H^+ from the surrounding intracellular medium for each mmol of acetate. The H^+ derives from either acidified, non-volatile buffers, primarily protein, or from H_2CO_3 derived from hydration of CO_2 originating in the citric acid cycle (Figure 1.2). Therefore, the uptake of H^+ in this reaction either restores acidified intracellular non-volatile buffer anion or results in de-novo generation of HCO_3^- buffer. The bulk of H^+ taken up derives from H_2CO_3 and a substantial portion of the HCO_3^- generated is promptly lost across the dialyser. Following conversion to acetyl-CoA, acetate will enter the Krebs cycle and be metabolized to CO_2 and water as outlined above (Figure 1.2). However, increased concentrations of acetyl-CoA are known to induce synthesis of oxaloacetate from pyruvate[72]. Pyruvate levels fall during acetate dialysis[73]. If these pathways become overloaded, acetyl-CoA will be diverted into the production of acetoacetate and β-hydroxybutyrate (Figure 1.4). Levels of acetoacetate and β-hydroxybutyrate have been shown to increase during acetate dialysis[68,71,74], suggesting that the capacity of the Krebs cycle to metabolize acetate is exceeded during acetate dialysis. Small increases in acetoacetate and β-hydroxybutyrate are also seen during bicarbonate dialysis[68]. This is attributed to the small amounts of acetate (2–8 mmol/L) contained in bicarbonate dialysate. Another important consideration in intermediary metabolism is the presence or absence of glucose in the dialysate. If absent from the dialysate, glucose will be lost from the blood, stimulating glycogenolysis and gluconeo-

19

genesis. The relative roles of gluconeogenesis and glycogenolysis in glucose replacement depend on the state of the glycogen stores. Gluconeogenesis from lactate involves the conversion of pyruvate to oxaloacetate. Ketone body production is sensitive to the glucagon–insulin ratio. The omission of glucose from the dialysate leads to a decrease in insulin levels and thus enhanced ketogenesis. This mechanism will exacerbate the production of acetoacetate and β-hydroxybutyrate.

The organic anions which accumulate during acetate dialysis are bicarbonate precursors and are removed from the blood during dialysis. Thus, the total H^+ removed during acetate dialysis is equal to the magnitude of body buffer repleted, which, in turn, is equal to the total acetate flux into the body minus the total HCO_3^- and organic anions lost across the dialyser (Figure 1.6). The differences in organic anion production between acetate and bicarbonate dialysis may be small; however, with high-efficiency dialysers and shorter duration of dialysis, this difference may become important. Net acid production remains unchanged but the bidirectional fluxes of bicarbonate and acetate will increase causing greater production and loss of acetoacetate and β-hydroxybutyrate. This may serve to decrease base repletion.

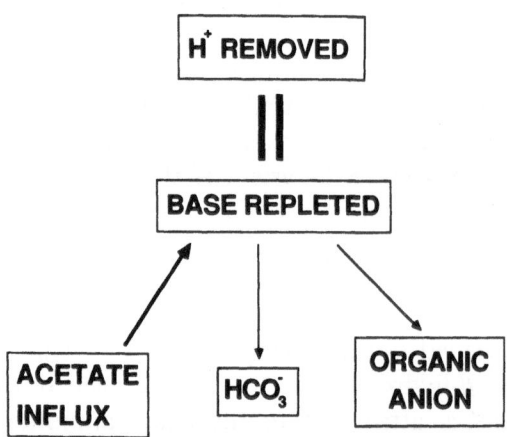

FIGURE 1.6 The amount of base repleted during acetate dialysis is a function of the amount of bicarbonate and organic anion lost in addition to the amount of acetate gained

In the case of bicarbonate dialysis, the amount of body buffer repleted (or H^+ removed) is equal to the total HCO_3^- flux into the body from the dialysate. The magnitude of the HCO_3^- flux will depend on the dialysate-to-blood concentration gradient, ultrafiltration rate and dialysance of the dialyser (Figure 1.7).

The concept that the net generation of base with acetate dialysis is insufficient to neutralize the interdialytic acid production, leading to gradual depletion of body buffer (e.g. bone[75]), is controversial. Recent studies have shown that substitution of bicarbonate for acetate leads to greater base repletion as judged by higher blood pH and bicarbonate levels (pre- and post-dialysis[68]) and a gradual repletion of buffer stores[67]. However, other workers have failed to show such differences[14,31,70].

In summary, bicarbonate dialysis has not been shown to be superior

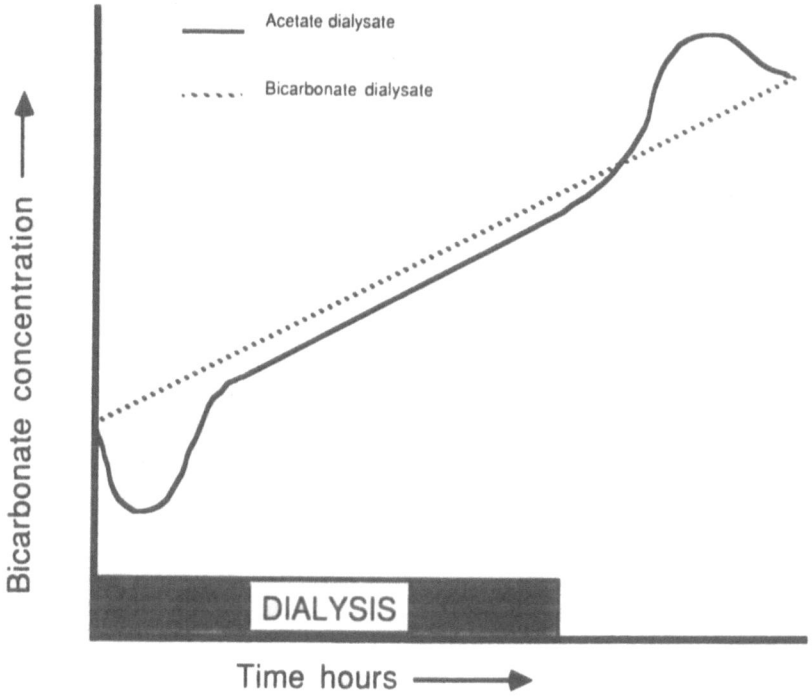

FIGURE 1.7 Change in bicarbonate concentration with time during acetate and bicarbonate dialysis

to acetate in the correction of chronic metabolic acidosis.

HYPERLIPOPROTEINAEMIA

Lipid abnormalities are present in over two thirds of patients with chronic renal failure undergoing haemodialysis[76]. The predominant abnormality is hypertriglyceridaemia with high levels of very-low-density lipoprotein (VLDL); in addition, there are reduced levels of the cholesterol fraction of high-density lipoprotein (HDL). The major cause of the abnormality is impaired removal of VLDL[77] due to reduced activity of lipoprotein lipase (LPL)[78,79], which, in turn, may be secondary to apoprotein C II deficiency in HDL, or an inhibitor of LPL in uraemic serum[80].

It has been postulated[81,82] that, since acetate is a substrate for lipid metabolism, the use of acetate in haemodialysis fluid, resulting in the delivery of more than 200 mmol/h of acetate to a dialysis patient, may exacerbate the lipid abnormalities and hence the accelerated atherosclerosis seen in dialysis patients.

Davidson and co-workers[83,84] looked at the fate of ^{14}C acetate during infusions in dogs and haemodialysis in humans. They showed that 1–2% of the infused load acetate was incorporated into lipid fractions. A figure of between 7–8% was achieved by Tolchin et al.[85]. Several studies have been performed looking at lipid levels during acetate dialysis and at changes in lipid levels with change from acetate to bicarbonte dialysis[17,75,86–90]. There are only two studies which have suggested an improvement in lipid profile with bicarbonate dialysis. Ahmad et al.[86] used extremely small numbers, did not use appropriate controls and some of the patients had unusually low triglyceride levels. Kluge et al.[87], in an abstract, described falling triglyceride levels during bicarbonate dialysis, with increases in LDL-Apo B, the HDL tri-glyceride fraction and HDL-Apo A1. The results of these two studies contradict a large number of well-conducted trials[17,75,88–90] which have consistently failed to show any improvement in lipid profiles with the use of bicarbonate dialysate.

Currently, the body of evidence suggests that the abnormal lipid profile seen in haemodialysis patients is an extension of that seen in patients with chronic renal failure prior to dialysis. The abnormality

22

is a result of impaired removal, rather than increased production, and is not corrected by the use of bicarbonate dialysate.

CONCLUSIONS

The description by Mion et al.[9] of the use of acetate as a dialysate buffer was undoubtedly a landmark in haemodialysis. Since the paper of Novello et al.[11], the debate has raged as to the benefits of bicarbonate over acetate and to the role of acetate in dialysis-related morbidity. Despite a large volume of work, many questions remain unanswered and others have been posed. Further work is required on several aspects, such as acetaldehyde metabolism, adenosine production and any possible interaction between new drugs, such as the HMG CoA reductase inhibitors, and acetate metabolism.

Nevertheless, the use of bicarbonate haemodialysis has increased dramatically in the last five years (Figure 1.8), so that, by the end of 1986, almost one-fifth of over 80 000 patients on haemodialysis in

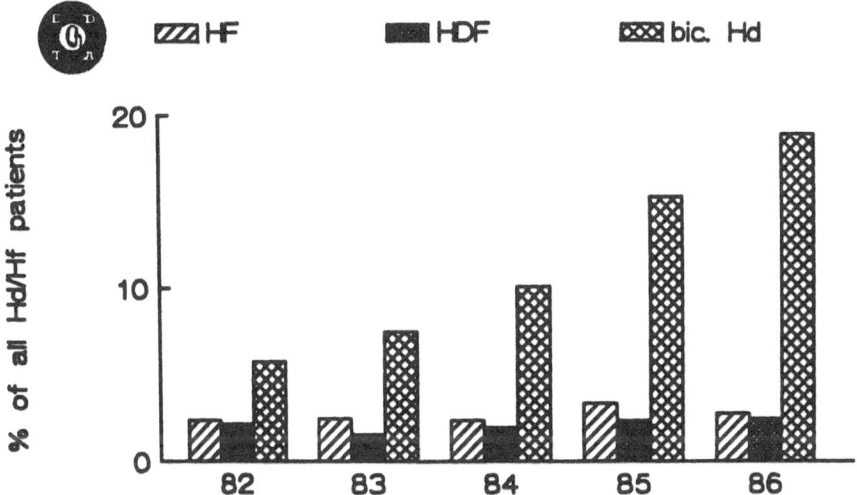

FIGURE 1.8 Proportion of patients treated by haemofiltration (HF), haemodiafiltration (HDF) and bicarbonate haemodialysis (bic. Hd) at the end of the years 1982–86 based on data from the centre EDTA questionnaire

Europe were on this form of therapy[91]. In Belgium, The Federal Republic of Germany, France, The German Democratic Republic and Italy, over 25% of haemodialysis patients were reported to be treated in this manner [see Table 1.4]. The proportion in the United Kingdom was much lower (7%). In Japan, the proportion was 58%, representing 42 340 haemodialysis patients on bicarbonate therapy in that country alone[92].

Reasons for the swing towards bicarbonate haemodialysis appear to be partly the employment of large-surface-area high-flux membrane dialysers in short dialysis schedules, and partly the acceptance for treatment of an increasing proportion of elderly and diabetic patients with vascular instability. The new fashion has been accelerated by commercial advertising. Patient pressure also probably contributes to the trend because patients are always eager to opt for ever shorter dialysis sessions and to grasp at any new technology which purports to reduce dialysis-associated morbidity.

The cost of bicarbonate haemodialysis for renal replacement therapy is about £500 per annum above the cost of conventional acetate haemodialysis. This extra cost is incurred by a higher price of the proportioning module, service costs and the cost of the bicarbonate concentrate. The higher cost could be justified in economic terms if it permitted the shortening of dialysis schedules and therefore the treatment of more patients in a given facility. However, it does not appear that such a gain is currently being achieved. The use of bicarbonate dialysis is more frequently justified in terms of the clinical needs of individual patients.

In 1983, Mansell and Wing[93] suggested guide-lines for the choice of patients for bicarbonate dialysis. Leunissen and Van Hoof[94] have formulated these guide-lines as a decision tree for the selection of patients who either demonstrate that they are, or can be predicted to be, vulnerable to acetate dialysis. Thus there may be a benefit in using bicarbonate dialysis for critically ill patients, for elderly patients with lung disease or ischaemic heart disease and for patients of any age with compromised left ventricular function. It is more debatable whether the 20% of parients who are slow metabolizers of acetate and develop high levels during acetate dialysis should be switched to bicarbonate dialysis. Patients with a slow metabolic rate for acetate do not necessarily have physiological intolerance. Proof that these

24

TABLE 1.4   The proportion (%) of haemodialysis patients treated by bicarbonate haemodialysis on 31 December 1986 in countries which reported to the EDTA Registry. Those countries which treated over 1000 patients by haemodialysis are shown individually and the total for the whole Registry is also shown

Country	Patients on haemodialysis	Patients on bicarbonate dialysis	Percentage
Austria	1 506	306	20
Belgium	2 350	994	42
Bulgaria	1 110	0	0
Czechoslovakia	1 164	33	3
Fed. Rep. Germany	16 727	4290	26
France	12 407	3157	25
German Dem. Rep.	1 883	557	30
Greece	1 251	14	1
Italy	13 400	3632	27
Netherlands	2 036	426	21
Poland	1 094	36	3
Portugal	2 011	13	1
Spain	8 152	904	11
Switzerland	1 174	205	17
United Kingdom	4 004	281	7
Yugoslavia	3 828	158	4
All other countries	6 449	368	6
Total Registry	80 546	15 374	19

patients are particularly prone to circulatory instability on acetate dialysis is lacking.

Claims for the benefit of bicarbonate dialysis should be viewed critically in the light of the evidence presented in this chapter. The extra cost of this form of dialysis should stimulate more critical evaluation of its role.

REFERENCES

1. Graham, T. (1861). Liquid diffusion applied to analysis. *Philos. Trans. R. Soc. London,*
2. Abell, J. J., Rowntree, L. C. and Turner, B. B. (1913). On the removal of diffusable substances from the circulating blood by means of dialysis. *Trans. Assoc. Am. Physicians*, **28**, 51
3. Haas, G. (1935). Die methoden der blutauswaschung (Methods of cleansing of blood). *Abderhaldens's Handb. Biol. Arbeitsmethoden,* **8**, 717 (in German)
4. Kolff, W. J. (1946). De Kunstmatige Nier (The Artificial Kidney). *MD thesis*, University of Groningen, The Netherlands, Kampen, JH Kok NV (in Dutch)
5. Kolff, W. J. (1947). *New Ways of Treating Ureamia.* (London: J. & A. Churchill)
6. Murray, G., Delorme, E. and Thomas, N. (1948). Artificial Kidney. *J. Am. Med. Assoc.* **137**, 1596
7. Alwall, N. (1947). On the artificial kidney. 1. Apparatus for dialysis of the blood in vivo. *Acta Med. Scand.,* **128**, 317
8. Skeggs, L. T. and Leonards, J. R. (1948). Studies on an artificial kidney. 1. Preliminary results with a new type of dialyser. *Science,* **108**, 212
9. Mion, C. M., Hegstrom, R. M., Boen, S. T. and Scribner, B. H. (1964). Substitution of sodium acetate for sodium bicarbonate in the bath fluid for haemodialysis. *Trans. Am. Soc. Artif. Intern. Organs*, **10**, 110–113
10. Lundquist, F. (1962). Production and utilization of free acetate in man. *Nature (London)*, **193**, 579
11. Novello, A., Kelsch, R. C. and Easterling, R. E. (1976). Acetate intolerance during haemodialysis. *Clin. Nephrol.* **5** (1), 29–32
12. Graefe, U., Milutinovich, J., Follette, W. C., Vizzo, J. E., Babb, A. L. and Schribner, B. H. (1978). Less dialysis induced mortality and vascular instability with bicarbonate in dialysate. *Ann. Intern. Med.,* **88**, 332–336
13. Patel, R., Ansari, A., Martin, C. and Funtinella, P. (1982). Bicarbonate and acetate metabolism during haemodialysis. *Contemp. Dial.,* **(1)**, 38–42
14. Bijaphala, S., Bell, A. J., Bennett, C. A., Evans, S. M. and Dawborn, J. K. (1985). Comparison of high and low sodium bicarbonate and acetate dialysis in stable chronic haemodialysis patients. *Clin. Nephrol.,* **23**, 179–183
15. Hakin, R. M., Pontzer, M-A., Tilton, D., Lazarus, M. and Gottlieb, M. N. (1985). Effects of acetate and bicarbonate in stable chronic dialysis patients. *Kidney Int.,* **28**, 535–540
16. Velez, R. L., Woodward, T. D. and Henrich, W. L. (1984). Acetate and bicarbonate haemodialysis in patients with and without autonomic dysfunction. *Kidney Int.,* **26**, 59–64
17. Man, N. K., Fornier, G., Thireau, P., Gaillard, J. L. and Funk-Brentano, J. L. (1982). Effect of bicarbonate-containing dialysate on chronic haemodialysis patients: a comparative study. *Int. Soc. Artif. Intern. Organs,* Nov. 421–425
18. Van Stone, J. C. and Cook, J. (1978). The effect of replacing acetate with bicarbonate in the dialysate of stable chronic haemodialysis patients. *Proc. Dial. Transplant Forum,* **8**, 103–105
19. Uldall, P. R., Kennedy, I., Craske, H., Porrett, E., Aid, J., Woods, F. and Levine, D. (1980). A double blind controlled trial of acetate versus bicarbonate dialysate. *Proc. Dial. Transplant Forum,* **10**, 220–223

20. Klopp, H., Wolfgruber, M., Pustelnik, A., Schiller, R., Hanefeld, F. and Kessel. (1982). Advantages of bicarbonate dialysis. *Artif. Organs*, **6** (4), 410–416
21. Pagel, M. D., Ahamen, S., Vizzo, J. E. and Schribner, B. H. (1982). Acetate and bicarbonate fluctuations and acetate intolerance during dialysis. *Kidney Int.*, **21**, 513–518
22. Boquin, E., Parnell, S., Grondin, G., Wollard, C., Leonard, D., Michaels, R. and Levin, N. W. (1977). Crossover study of the effects of different dialysate sodium concentrations in large surface area, short term dialysis. *Proc. Dial. Transplant Forum*, **7**, 48
23. Van Stone, J. C. and Cooke, J. C. (1978). Decreased post dialysis fatigue with increased dialysate sodium concentration. *Proc. Dial. Transplant Forum*, **8**, 152
24. Ogden, D. A. (1978). A double-blind crossover comparison of high and low sodium dialysis. *Proc. Dial. Transplant Forum*, **8**, 157
25. Port, F. K., Johnson, W. J. and Klass, D. W. (1973). Prevention of dialysis disequilibrium syndrome by use of high sodium concentration in the dialysate. *Kidney Int.*, **3**, 327
26. Shimizu, A. G., Taylor, D. W., Sackett, D. L., Smith, E. K. M., Barnes, C. C., Hoda, P., Lennox, G., Martin, J., McNeaney, H., Mukherjee, J. and Uniyal, B. (1983). Reducing patient morbidity from high efficiency haemodialysis: A double blind cross-over trial. *Trans. Am. Soc. Artif. Intern. Organs*, **29**, 666–668
27. Kveim, M. and Bredese, J. E. (1979). A gas chromatographic method for determination of acetate levels in body fluids. *Clin. Chim. Acta*, **92**, 27–32
28. Mansell, M. A., Nunan, T. O., Laker, M. F., Boon, N. A. and Wing, A. J. (1979). Incidence and significance of rising blood acetate levels during haemodialysis. *Clin. Nephrol.*, **12** (1), 22–25
29. Weiner, M. W. (1979). Acetate metabolism during haemodialysis. *Artif. Organs*, **6** (4), 370–377
30. Mansell, M. A., Morgan, S. H., Moore, R., Kong, C. H., Laker, M. F. and Wing, A. J. (1987). Cardiovascular and acid–base effects of acetate and bicarbonate haemodialysis. *Nephrol. Dial. Transplant.*, **1**, 229–232
31. Cairns, H. S., Rideout, J. M., Peters, T. J., Laker, M. F. and Mansell, M. A. (1988). Changes in blood acetaldehyde concentrations during haemodialysis. *Nephrol. Dial. Transplant.* (In press)
32. Kirkendol, P. L., Devia, C. J., Bower, J. D. and Holbert, R. D. (1977). A comparison of the cardiovascular effects of sodium acetate, sodium bicarbonate and other potential sources of fixed base in haemodialysate solutions. *Trans. Am. Soc. Artif. Intern. Organs*, **23**, 399
33. Aizawa, Y., Ohmori, T., Imai, Y., Matsuoka, M. and Hirasawa, Y. (1977). Depressant effect of acetate upon the human cardiovascular system. *Clin. Nephrol.*, **8** (5), 477–480
34. Kirkendol, P. L., Robie, N. W., Gonzalez, F. M. and Devia, C. J. (1978). Cardiac and vascular effects of infused sodium acetate in dogs. *Trans. Am. Soc. Artif. Intern. Organs*, **24**, 714–718
35. Chen, T. S., Friedman, H. S., Dell Monte, M. and Smith, A. J. (1979). Haemodynamic changes during dialysis. *Proc. Clin. Dial. Transplant. Forum*, **9**, 66
36. Iseki, K., Onoyama, K., Maeda, T., Shimamatsu, K., Harada, A., Fulimi, S. and Omae, T. (1980). Comparison of haemodynamics induced by conventional acetate haemodialysis, bicarbonate haemodialysis and ultrafiltration. *Clin. Nephrol.*, **14** (6), 294–298

37. Cannella, G., Cancarini, G., De Marinis, S., Maccagnola, V. and Maiorca, R. (1982). Interrelationships between blood pressure, blood gases and plasma acetate during conventional haemodialysis. *Int. J. Artif. Organs*, **5** (6), 357–360
38. Nitenberg, A., Huyghebaert, M-F., Blanchet, F. and Amiel, C. (1984). Analysis of increased myocardial contractility during sodium acetate infusion in humans. *Kidney Int.*, **26**, 744–751
39. Wehle, B., Asaba, H., Castenfors, J., Furst, P., Grahn, A., Gunnarsson, B., Shaldon, S. and Bergstrom, J. (1978). The influence of dialysis fluid composition on the blood pressure response during dialysis. *Clin. Nephrol.*, **10**(2), 62–66
40. Nixon, J. V., Mitchell, J. H. and McPhaul, J. J. (1983). Effects of haemodialysis on left ventricular function. *J. Clin. Invest.*, **71**, 377–384
41. Mansell, M. A., Crowther, A., Laker, M. F. and Wing, A. J. (1982). The effects of hyperacetataemia on cardiac output during regular haemodialysis. *Clin. Nephrol.*, **18**(3), 130–134
42. Shick, E. C., Idelson, B. A., Liang, C., Redline, R. C. and Bernard, D. B. (1983). Comparison of the haemodynamic response to haemodialysis with acetate or bicarbonate. *Trans. Am. Soc. Artif. Intern. Organs*, **29**, 25–28
43. Chen, T. S., Friedman, H. S., Smith, A. J. and Del Monte, M. L. (1983). Haemodynamic changes during haemodialysis: role of dialysate. *Clin. Nephrol.*, **20**(4), 190–196
44. Mehta, B. R., Fischer, D., Ahmad, M. and Dubose, T. D. (1983). Effects of acetate and bicarbonate haemodialysis on cardiac function in chronic dialysis patients. *Kidney Int.*, **24**, 782-787
45. Ruder, M. A., Alpert, M. A., Van Stone, J., Selmon, M. R., Kelly, D. L., Haynie, J. D. and Perkins, S. K. (1985). Comparative effects of acetate and bicarbonate haemodialysis on left ventricular function. *Kidney Int.*, **27**, 768–773
46. Henrich, W. L., Woodard, T. D., Meyer, B. D., Chappell, T. R. and Rubin, L. J. (1983). High sodium bicarbonate and acetate haemodialysis: Double blind crossover comparison of haemodynamic and ventilatory effects. *Kidney Int.*, **24**, 240–245
47. Borges, H. F., Fryd, D. S., Rosa, A. A. and Kyellstrand, C. M. (1981). Hypotension during acetate and bicarbonate dialysis in patients with acute renal failure. *Am. J. Nephrol.*, **1**, 24–30
48. Vincente, J-L., Vanherweghem, J-L., Degaute, J-P., Berre, J., Dufaye, P. and Kahn, R. L. (1982). Acetate-induced myocardial depression during haemodialysis for acute renal failure. *Kidney Int.* **22**, 653–657
49. Huyghebaert, M-F., Dhainaut, J-M., Monsallier, J. F. and Schlemmer, B. (1985). Bicarbonate haemodialysis of patients with acute renal failure and severe sepsis. *Crit. Care Med.*, **13**(10), 840
50. Leunissen, K. M. L., Hoorntje, S. J., Fiers, H. A., Dekkers, W. T. and Mulder, A. W. (1986). Acetate versus bicarbonate haemodialysis in critically ill patients. *Nephron*, **42**, 146–151
51. Johnson, N. R., Bischel, M. D. and Boylen, C. T. (1970). Hypoxaemia and hyperventilation in chronic haemodialysis (abstract). *Clin. Res.*, **19**, 145
52. Leenen, F. H. H., Buda, A. J., Smith, D. L., Farrel, S., Levine, D. Z. and Uldall, P. R. (1984). Haemodynamic changes during acetate and bicarbonate haemodialysis. *Artif. Organs*, **8**(4), 411–417
53. Ahmad, S., Pagel, M., Shen, F., Vizzo, J. and Schribner, B. H. (1981). The role of hypoxaemia in the expression of acetate intolerance. *Kidney Int.*, **19**, 140

54. Bischel, M. D., Orrell, F. L., Scoles, B. G., Mohler, J. G. and Barbour, B. H. (1973). Effects of microemboli blood filtration during haemodialysis. *Trans. Am. Soc. Artif. Intern. Organs,* **19,** 492–497
55. Craddock, P. R., Feher, J., Brigham, K. L., Kronenberg, R. S. and Jacob, H. J. (1977). Complement and leucocyte-mediated pulmonary dysfunction in haemodialysis. *N. Engl. J. Med.,* **296,** 769–774
56. Sherlock, J., Ledwith, J. and Letteri, J. (1977). Hypoventilation and hypoxaemia during haemodialysis. *Trans. Am. Soc. Artif. Intern. Organs,* **23,** 406–410
57. Oh, M. S., Uribarri, J., Del Monte, M. L., Heneghan, W. F., Kee, C. S., Friedman, E. A. and Carroll, H. J. (1985). A mechanism of hypoxaemia during haemodialysis. *Am. J. Nephrol.,* **5,** 366–371
58. Craddock, P. R., Fehr, J., Dalmasso, A. P., Brigham, L. and Jacob, H. S. (1977). Haemodialysis leucopenia: pulmonary vascular leucostasis resulting from complement activation by dialyser cellophane membranes. *J. Clin. Invest.,* **59,** 879–888
59. Dumler, F. and Levin, N. W. (1979). Leucopenia and hypoxaemia. Unrelated effects of dialysis. *Arch. Intern. Med.,* **139,** 1103–1106
60. Jacob, A. I., Gavellas, G., Zarco, R., Perez, G. and Bourgoignie, J. J. (1980). Leucopenia, hypoxia, and complement function with different haemodialysis membranes. *Kidney Int.,* **18,** 505–509
61. Brautbar, N., Shinaberger, J. H., Millar, J. H. and Nachman, M. (1980). Haemodialysis hypoxaemia: evaluation of mechanisms utilizing sequential ultrafiltration dialysis. *Nephron,* **26,** 96–99
62. Igarashi, H., Kioi, S., Gejyo, F. and Arakawa, M. (1985). Physiological approach to dialysis-induced hypoxaemia. *Nephron,* **41,** 62–69
63. Carlon, G. C., Campfield, P. B., Goldiner, P. L. and Turnbull, A. D. (1979). Hypoxaemia during dialysis. *Crit. Care Med.,* **71,** 497–499
64. Raja, R. M., Kramer, M. S., Rosenbaum, J. L., Bolisay, C. G. and Krug, M. J. (1981). Haemodialysis associated hypoxaemia. Role of acetate and pH in etiology. *Trans. Am. Soc. Artif. Intern. Organs,* **27,** 180–183
65. Dolan, M. J., Whipp, B. J., Davidson, W. D., Weitzman, R. E. and Wasserman, K. (1981). Hypopnoea associated with acetate haemodialysis: carbon dioxide-flow-dependent ventilation. *N. Engl. J. Med.,* **305,** 72–75
66. Oh, M., Uribarri, J. V., Del Monte, M., Friedman, M. and Caroll, H. (1979). Consumption of CO_2 in metabolism of acetate as an explanation for hypoventilation and hypoxaemia during haemodialysis. (Abstract) *Kidney Int.,* **16,** 895
67. Ward, R. A., Wathen, R. L. and Williams, T. E. (1982). Effects of long-term bicarbonate haemodialysis on acid base status. *Trans. Am. Soc. Artif. Intern. Organs,* **28,** 295–298
68. Ward, R. A., Wathen, R. L., Williams, T. E. and Harding, G. B. (1987). Haemodialysate composition and intradialytic metabolism, acid–base and potassium changes. *Kidney Int.,* **32,** 129–135
69. Brenes, L. G., Brenes, J. N. and Hernandez, M. M. (1977). Familial proximal renal tubular acidosis. A distinct clinical entity. *Am. J. Med.,* **63,** 244–252
70. Brezin, J. H., Schwartz, A. B. and Chinitz, J. L. (1985). Switch from acetate to bicarbonate dialysis: Better dialysis tolerance but failure to improve acidosis and hypertriglyceridaemia. *Trans. Am. Soc. Artif. Intern. Organs,* **31,** 343–348
71. Vreman, H. J., Assomull, V. M., Kaiser, B. A., Blaschke, T. F. and Weiner, M. W. (1980). Acetate metabolism and acid–base homeostasis during haemodialysis: Influence of dialyser efficiency and rate of acetate metabolism. *Kidney Int.,* **18** (suppl. 10), S62–S74

72. Keech, D. B. and Utter, M. F. (1963). Pyruvate carboxylase. II. Properties. *J. Biol. Chem.*, **238**, 2609–2614
73. Kaiser, B. A., Potter, D. E., Bryant, R. E., Vreman, H. J. and Weiner, M. W. (1981). Acid–base changes and acetate metabolism during routine and high-efficiency haemodialysis in children. *Kidney Int.*, **19**, 70–79
74. Wathen, R. L., Keshaviah, P., Hommeyer, P., Cadwell, K. and Comty, C. M. (1978). The metabolic effects of haemodialysis with and without glucose in the dialysate. *Am. J. Clin. Nutr.*, **31**, 1870–1875
75. Kobayashi, N., Okubo, M., Marumo, F. and Jakamura, H. (1983). Effects of dialysis on lipid metabolism in chronic renal failure – acetate versus bicarbonate. *Int. J. Artif. Organs*, **64**, 187–190
76. Ibels, L. S., Simons, L. A., King, J. O., Williams, P. F., Neale, F. C. and Stewart, J. H. (1975). Studies on the nature and causes of hyperlipidaemia in uraemia, maintenance dialysis and renal transplantation. *Q. J. Med.*, **44**, 601
77. Cattran, D. C., Steiner, G., Fenten, S. S. A. and Wilson, D. R. (1974). Hyper-triglyceridaemia in uraemia and the use of triglyceridaemia turnover to define pathogenesis. *Trans. Am. Soc. Artif. Intern. Organs*, **20-A**, 148
78. Ibels, L. S., Reardon, M. F. and Nestel, P. J. (1976). Plasma post-heparin lipolytic activity and triglyceride clearance in uraemic haemodialysis patients and renal allograft recipients. *J. Lab. Clin. Med.*, **87**, 648
79. Chan, M., Varghese, Z., Persand, J., Baillod, R. and Moorhead, J. (1982). Hyperlipidaemia in patients on maintenance haemodialysis and peritoneal dialysis: the relative roles of triglyceride production and triglyceride removal. *Clin. Nephrol.*, **17**, 183–190
80. Hueck, C. and Ritz, E. (1980). Hyperlipoproteinaemia in renal insufficiency. *Nephron*, **25**, 1–7.
81. Gonzalez, F. M., Pearson, J. E., Garbus, S. B. and Holbert, R. D. (1974). On the effects of acetate during haemodialysis. *Trans. Am. Soc. Artif. Intern. Organs*, **20-A**, 169
82. Tsaltas, T. T. and Friedman, E. A. (1980). Plasma lipid studies of uraemic patients during haemodialysis. *Am. J. Clin. Nutr.*, **21**, 430
83. Rorke, S. J., Davidson, W. D., Guo, S. S. and Morin, R. J. (1977). The fate of ^{14}C acetate during dialysis. *Proc. Eur. Dial. Transplant. Assoc.*, **14**, 394
84. Morin, R. J., Guo, S. S., Rorke, S. J. and Davidson, W. D. (1978). Lipid metabolism in uraemic and non-uraemic dogs during and after haemodialysis with acetate. *J. Dial.*, **2**, 113
85. Tolchin, N., Roberts, J. L., Hayashi, J. and Lewis, E. J. (1977). Metabolic consequences of high mass transfer haemodialysis. *Kidney Int.*, **11**, 366
86. Ahmad, S., Haas, L., Pagel, M. and Sherrard, D. (1980). Improved lipid profiles with bicarbonate dialysis. *Proc. Dial. Transplant Forum*, **10**, 186–189
87. Kluge, M., Wildberger, R., Hueck, C., Wirth, C. and Ritz, P. (1980). Effect on serum lipids of bicarbonate dialysis. (Abstract) *Kidney Int.*, **17**, 409
88. Assomull, V. M., Vreman, H. J. and Weiner, M. W. (1979). Evidence that acetate in dialysate does not stimulate lipid synthesis. *Proc. Dial. Transplant Forum*, **9**, 73–79
89. Savdie, E., Mahony, J. F. and Stewart, J. H. (1977). Effect of acetate on serum lipids in maintenance haemodialysis. *Trans. Am. Soc. Artif. Intern. Organs*, **23**, 385–392

90. Morin, R. J., Srikantaiah, M. V., Woodley, Z. and Davidson, W. D. (1980). Effects of haemodialysis with acetate vs. bicarbonate on plasma lipids and lipo-protein levels in uraemic patients. *J. Dial.*, **4**(1), 9–20

91. Broyer, M., Brunner, F. P., Brynger, H., Fassbinder, W., Geerlings, W., Rizzoni, G., Selwood, N. H., Tufveson, G. and Wing, A. J. (1986). *Combined Report on Regular Dialysis and Transplantation in Europe, XVII,* EDTA Registry, St Thomas' Hospital, London SE1 7EH

92. Odaka, M. for the *Japanese Society of Dialysis Therapy,* (1987). Chiba University of Japan

93. Mansell, M. A. and Wing, A. J. (1983). Acetate or bicarbonate for haemodialysis? *Br. Med. J.,* **287,** 308–309

94. Leunissen, K. M. L. and Van Hooff, J. P. (1988). Acetate or bicarbonate for haemodialysis? *Nephrol. Dial. Transplant.,* **3,** 1–7

2
HAEMOFILTRATION

A. M. MARTIN AND M. I. McHUGH

HAEMOFILTRATION: PRINCIPLES, MATERIALS AND EQUIPMENT

Principles

The term 'haemofiltration' was suggested by Burton in 1976[1]. It describes a process of blood purification first conceived by Henderson *et al.* in 1967[2]. The physical principal involved is convection where solute movement occurs with fluid flow, as illustrated in Figure 2.1. This differs from dialysis in which solute molecules pass through a

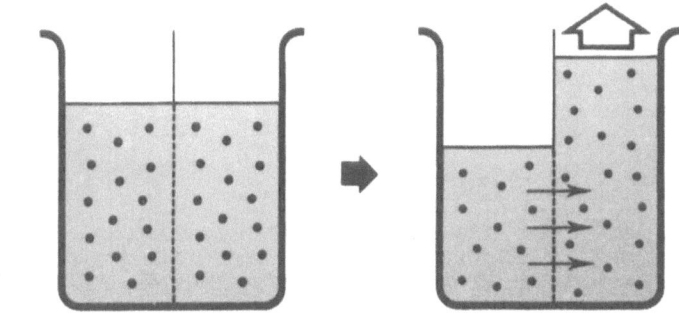

FIGURE 2.1   Convection: the movement of solutes with a water-flow, 'solvent-drag'; e.g. the movement of membrane-permeable solutes with ultrafiltered water

semipermeable membrane into an electrolyte solution by diffusion due to concentration gradient. A comparison of clearances in haemodialysis and haemofiltration is shown in Figure 2.2 and illustrates that clearance in haemofiltration is relatively independent of solute molecular weight (up to 10 000 Da).

Bulk flow is generated by a pressure difference across a membrane with hydraulic permeability (up to 50 × that of Cuprophan) to form a filtrate which is discarded. There is no dialysing fluid and, consequently, diffusion does not take place. Water and electrolytes are replaced, as required, into the blood circulation. The replacement fluid may be introduced before the membrane filter (predilution) or after the filter with the venous return into the circulation (postdilution). The predilution system requires larger amounts of replacement fluid. Theoretically this mode favours dissociation of partially protein-

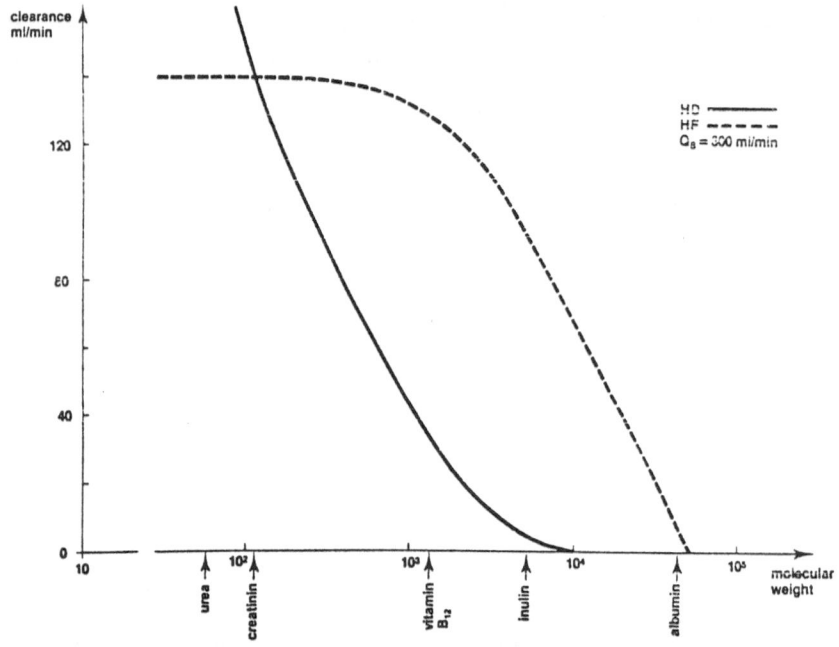

FIGURE 2.2   Clearance comparison

bound solutes and so increases solute removal. Predilution results in higher ultrafiltration flow rates and preserves the efficiency of the filter by minimizing protein layering. At present, postdilution is more widely used for reasons of cost.

Performance variables

The rate of convection is mainly influenced by transmembrane pressure (TMP), blood composition and membrane characteristics. Filter design can also be an important factor.

Transmembrane pressure

The initial slope of the filtration curve is linear, but gradually tails off due to the protein layering effect which is dependent upon blood composition.

Blood composition

Solute transport is affected by the adsorption of plasma protein molecules on to the membrane surface. Cells and the adsorbed protein form a secondary membrane leading to a reduction in ultrafiltration and convection as the treatment progresses. Any increase in blood protein concentration (Figure 2.3) reduces filtration. This secondary membrane can be reduced by increasing wall shear rates using high blood flows. Some workers have identified the shearing action of red blood cells as the most significant effect in reducing this layer[3]. Increasing the haematocrit reduces ultrafiltration rates[1].

Blood flow rates

The efficiency and duration of each treatment session depends on the blood flow rate (Q_B), the filter surface area and the exchange volume. The relationship between the ultrafiltration rate and the blood flow

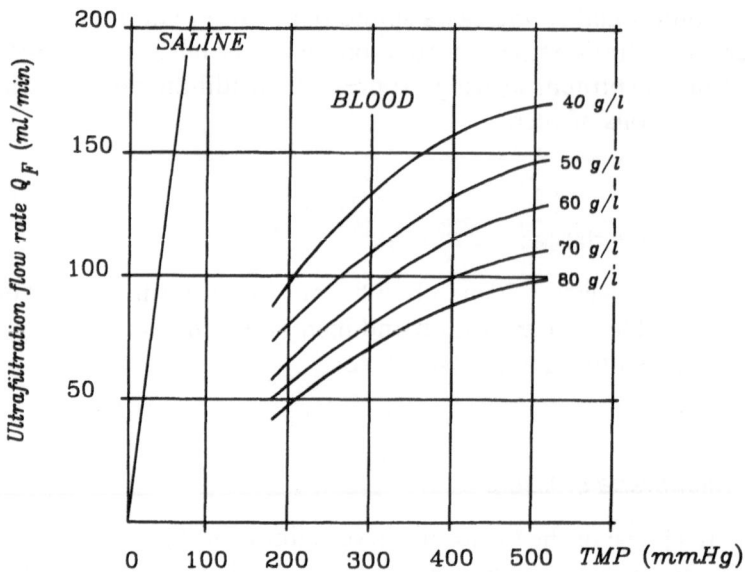

FIGURE 2.3   Ultrafiltration with Gambro FH77 varying protein
concentration
In vitro filtration with blood: Hct 25%; Q_B 300 ml/min temperature 37°C

rate for a polyamide filter is shown in Figure 2.4. The filtration rate
increases with surface area in a non-linear fashion, and, at blood flow
rates of 100 ml per minute, the same filtration rate is observed for
both small and large surface area devices. Significant improvement in
filtration rates for large surface area devices appears at blood flow
rates of 300 ml per minute or more.

Clearance calculation

The calculation of solute clearance during haemofiltration is based on
the sieving coefficient (S) which is the ratio of filtrate (Cf) to plasma
water (Cpw) solute concentrations. S = Cf/Cpw, an average plasma
water concentration being the mean of the arterial and the venous
plasma levels (Cpwa + Cpwv)/2. Clearance approximates to sieving
coefficient multiplied by ultrafiltration rate.

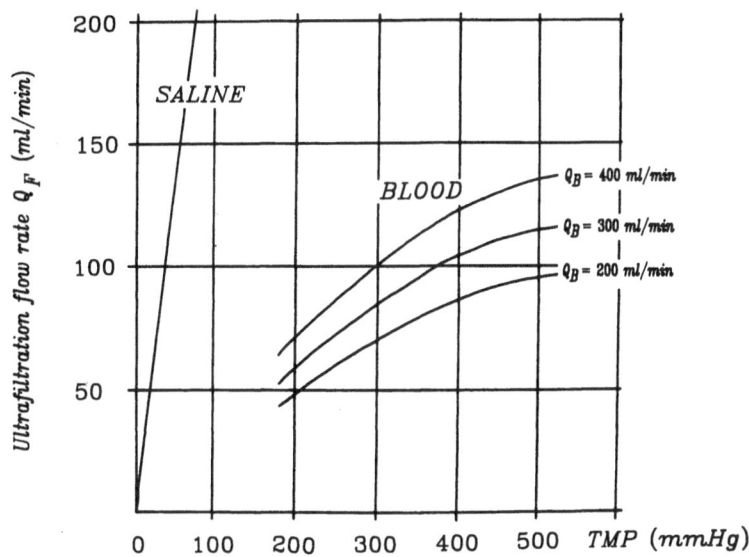

FIGURE 2.4   Ultrafiltration with Gambro FH77 varying blood flow rate
(Q_B)
In vitro filtration with bovine blood: Hct 25%; Pct 65 g/L; temperature 37°C

Materials

The characteristics required of a membrane for haemofiltration are
high plasma water permeability, impermeability to albumin, high
permeability to solutes smaller than plasma proteins and blood com-
patibility. Low protein adsorption and high mechanical strengths are
also desirable. The membranes are described as being finely porous
and made from hydrophilic gel polymers, such as cellulose acetate,
polyvinyl alcohol, polycarbonate polyether, polymethyl methacrylate,
or asymmetric polymers, such as polyamide, polysulphone and polyacrylonitrile. Typically, these asymmetric materials consist of a membrane skin about 0.1 μm thick on a sponge-like support about 65 μm
thick. The blood is exposed to the membrane skin aspect. Membranes
are formed in flat sheets or hollow fibres. The specifications of commercially available haemofiltration devices are given in Table 2.1. An
open view of a polyamide hollow fibre is illustrated in Figure 2.5.

TABLE 2.1 Specifications of widely used, commercially available haemofilters

Membrane material	Surface area range (m²)	Sterilization	Product name (manufacturer) and approx. cost
Polyamide (fibre)	0.16–1.95	ETO*	FH 22, 55, 66, 77, 88 (Gambro) £36–40
Polysulphone (fibre)	0.25–1.1	ETO	D 20a, 30a, 40 (Amicon) £45
Polyacrylonitrile (fibre)	1.10–2.0	ETO	Pan 150, 200, 250 (Asahi) £40
Polysulphone (fibre)	1.9	ETO	HF 80 (Fresenius) £45
Acrylonitrile and sodium methyl sulphonate (plate/fibre)	0.5–1.2	ETO/GAMMA**	Biospal 1200S–3000S (Hospal) £22–30
Cellulose triacetate (plate)	0.4–1.0	ETO	40041–40043 (Sartorius) £40

* Ethylene oxide
** Gamma radiation

Equipment

General description

By means of a pumped extracorporeal blood circuit, the system ultrafilters the blood through a membrane filter and accurately reconstitutes the blood volume by delivering substitution fluid. In Europe, the most widely used system is manufactured by Gambro and consists of the standard blood monitor to pump and control the arterial and venous circuit, a haemofiltration monitor, a haemofilter and the desired replacement fluid. A haemofiltration system and monitor are

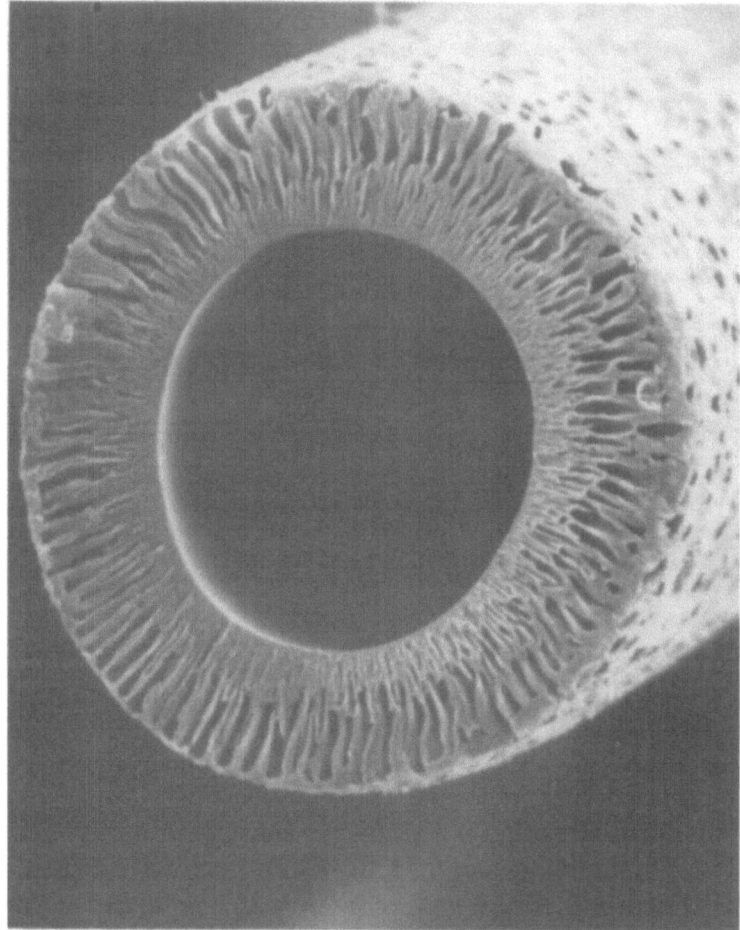

FIGURE 2.5   Polyamide hollow fibre (SEM view)

illustrated in Figures 2.6 and 2.7. It includes ultrafiltrate and infusate circuits, a weighing scale and data selection display panel.

Monitor function

The main function of the monitor is to control the amount of ultrafilt-rate drawn from the patient and the amount of replacement fluid given to the patient during the treatment. It is essentially a sophisticated

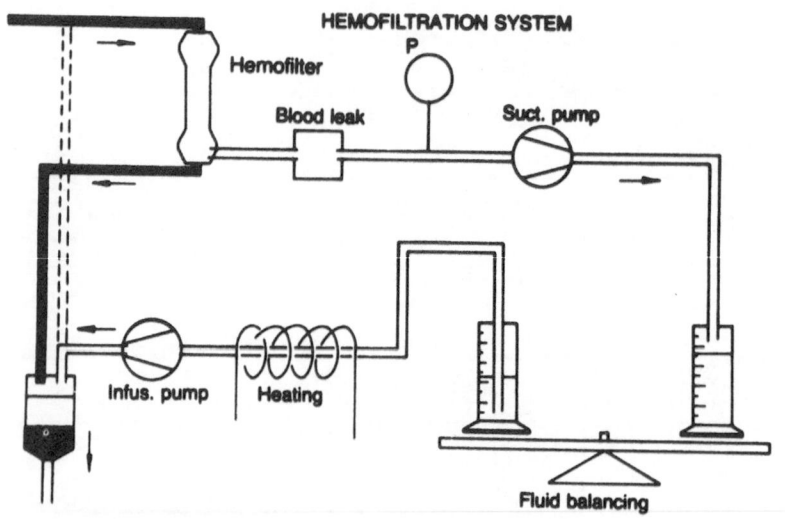

FIGURE 2.6 Haemofiltration system – schematic

microprocessor-controlled balancing system, which ensures accurate and linear weight loss. At the beginning of a treatment the desired weight loss, the amount of substitution fluid to be reinfused and the transmembrane pressure are set. The machine will then automatically carry out the treatment according to the pre-set values. Any significant deviation in the ultrafiltrate or infusate delivery results in an alarm situation. The machine continues to run and control the treatment automatically until the pre-set values are achieved. It is usual to exchange 20–30 L fluid during one treatment. Obviously, an increase in the fluid exchange volume permits a greater clearance of solutes. The length of treatment is governed by the filtration rate and a higher filtration rate will shorten the treatment time. The control of fluid handling by a fully automated machine contributes considerably to the safety and simplicity of a haemofiltration treatment.

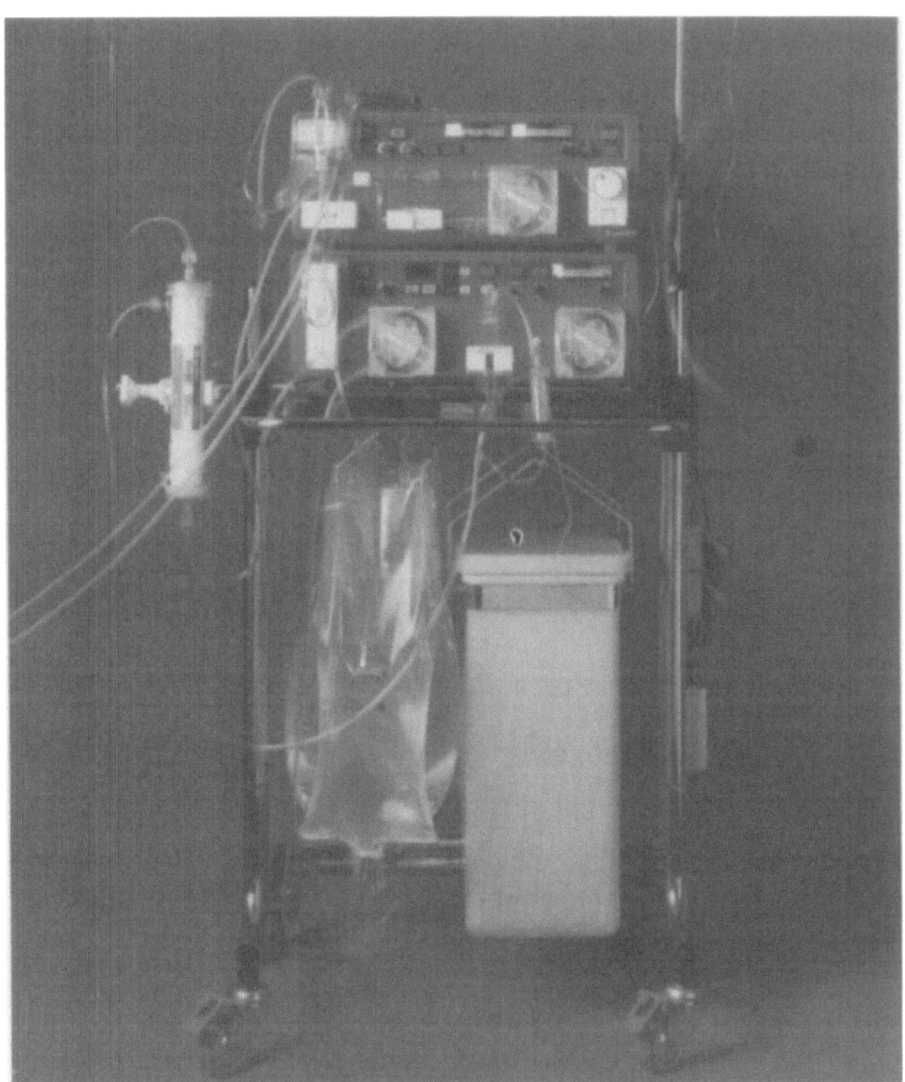

FIGURE 2.7   Haemofiltration system

Systems available

There are four systems in use in Europe (Gambro, Fresenius, Sartorius, designed for haemofiltration, and Braun, designed for high flux dialysis).

Continuous arterovenous haemofiltration (CAVH) developed as a treatment for uraemia from the work of Silverstein et al.[4] who incorporated ultrafiltration units into haemodialyser circuits and Henderson et al.[2] who proposed the technique of diafiltration as an alternative to dialysis. A CAVH circuit is illustrated in Figure 2.8. Comparisons of haemofiltration (HF) and CAVH are made in the section on acute renal failure.

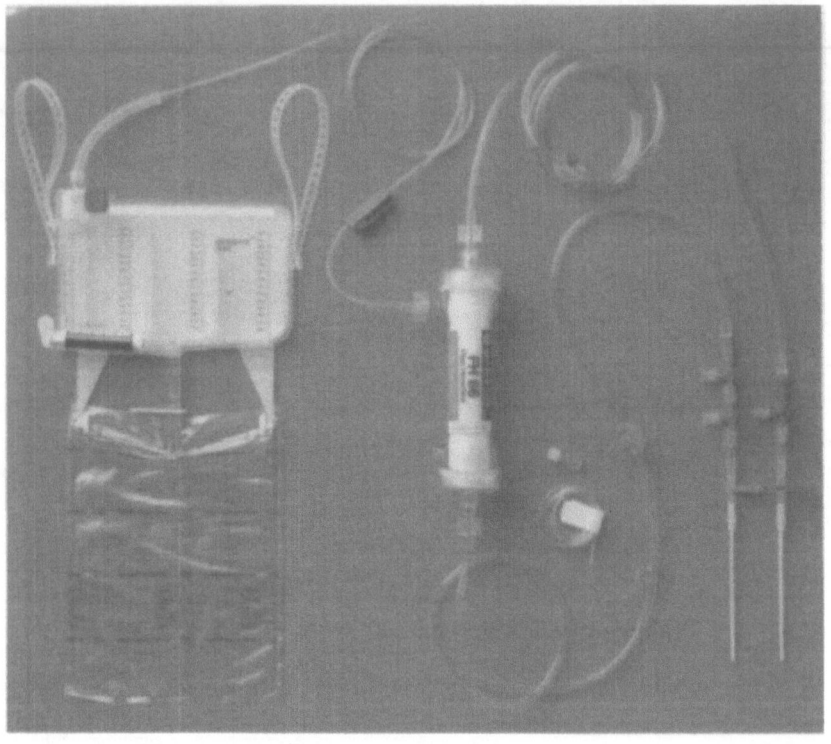

FIGURE 2.8   CAVH circuit

Staff training

The introduction of the new technology into clinical practice has been greatly facilitated by the establishment of a training course by Gambro. A study day programme describes the principles, range of techniques, future developments and provides 'hands on' experience in clinical use. These courses are provided free of charge to interested units.

HAEMOFILTRATION (HF) IN ACUTE RENAL FAILURE

Mortality in acute renal failure is now rarely a direct consequence of uraemia though morbidity may still be related to the dialysis process. Of importance in this respect is the need for improved haemodynamic stability and acid–base balance in patients with multisystem failure. Even small modifications in technique applied to renal, respiratory and cardiovascular assistance might lead to improved chances of survival. There are conflicting views as to whether intensive dialysis improves wound healing, infection control, nutritional state and overall survival[5-7]. Controlled trials are still required and should also be applied to filtration techniques, continuous arteriovenous haemofiltration (CAVH) and haemofiltration (HF).

CAVH

CAVH was originally devised as a means of ultrafiltration to enable fluid and nutritional requirements to be provided continuously, but has been adopted by some nephrologists and intensivists to treat uraemia continuously using ultrafiltration rates of about 14 L daily[8]. Golper[9] considers the ideal indications for CAVH in acute renal failure are in haemodynamically unstable patients or those who have a direct contraindication for acute peritoneal dialysis. He also cites diuretic unresponsive oliguria and 'bed-ridden' acute renal failure patients as suitable settings. This technique has, on occasions, been introduced into intensive care units when haemodialysis expertise and facilities were not available and intensivists should be aware of potential problems. A mistake in fluid balancing represents a risk; continuous heparinization can lead to problems if emergency surgery is required and bleeding sites are present; between 16 and 40% of patients have had bleeding complications[10]; the system does not satisfactorily deal with the hypercatabolic or hyperkalaemic patient; and, most importantly, CAVH demands close nurse supervision and a knowledge of problems associated with extracorporeal circulation.

The nephrologist and the renal nurse are in daily contact with unstable patients on dialysis and acquire skills in adapting the regime according to efficacy and complications. The intensive care nurse, however, does not have regular exposure to dialysis but has many other demands in relation to ventilation and nutrition.

One group reported that CAVH was associated with more clinical ill effects than haemodialysis (HD) when the differences in treatment efficiency were taken into consideration[10].

Haemofiltration

Haemofiltration (HF), used daily as an alternative to dialysis in conjunction with periods of continuous ultrafiltration as required, provides a treatment modality that does offer advantages over haemodialysis.

Vascular access

A radial Scribner shunt has, in our experience, provided the most satisfactory access in most cases of acute renal failure, enabling periods of continuous ultrafiltration to proceed after haemofiltration.

A 15 gauge vessel tip is the minimum required for adequate blood flow rates. Where radial access has not been possible, veno-venous cannulation, using a subclavian vein, is a suitable alternative but does not permit unpumped ultrafiltration to proceed between treatments.

With the advent of subclavian cannulation in acute renal failure, both the skill in inserting radial shunts and the vigilance of the nephrologist over potentially vital forearm vasculature has declined. The advent of haemofiltration necessitates a reversal of this trend.

TABLE 2.2 Cardiovascular events in patients with acute renal and respiratory failure treated by HF

	Dysrhythmia incidence	Dysrhythmias requiring therapy	Previous CVS disease	Cardiac cause of death
Survivors	7/11 (64%)	1 (14%)	3 (27%)	—
Non-survivors	12/16 (75%)	10 (83%)	5 (31%)	10 (83%)

Filter 're-use'

At the end of an HF treatment, the same filter can be incorporated into a continuous ultrafiltration circuit if required.

Cardiovascular stability

Cardiovascular deaths are common in patients with severe acute renal failure. Table 2.2. shows the relationship between cardiovascular events and outcome in a series of patients with acute renal and respiratory failure, treated in this unit over a four-year period. HF has been shown by others to result in improved cardiovascular stability over HD in uraemic patients[11]. In our experience, there is greater cardiovascular stability in critically ill patients. Despite the requirements of high blood flow rates (> 300 ml/min), ultrafiltration can proceed in some hypotensive patients as illustrated in Figure 2.9 in a patient presenting with acute renal and respiratory failure precipitated by acute haemorrhagic pancreatitis. The reason for such stability of blood pressure is not clear. Dialysis-induced hypotension occurs if the ultrafiltration rate exceeds vascular filling and if solutes are moved selectively to or from the extracellular fluid. Even sequential ultrafiltration does not prevent hypotonic circulatory reactions during dialysis. Blood cellulose membrane interactions can upset blood pressure early in the course of dialysis. Haemofilters consist of non-cellulose membranes and non-pyrogen-containing infusion fluids are used.

45

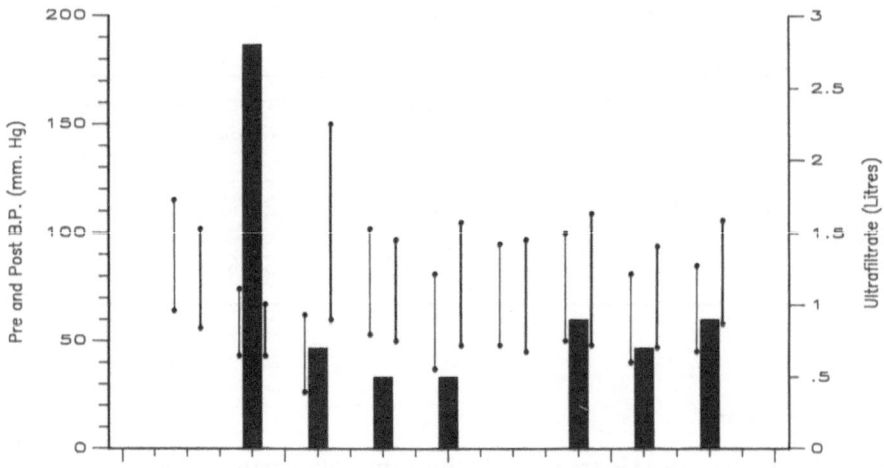

FIGURE 2.9   HF in the haemodynamically unstable patient (Q_B 300–400 ml/min)

Interleukin 1 production leading to PGE_2-induced vasodilatation is not a feature of these systems – unlike dialysis.

Acid–base control

Acetate buffers are used in haemodialysis and haemofiltration in similar quantities for each treatment. Higher blood bicarbonate levels have been consistently observed as a result of haemofiltration though the explanation is not clear[12].

HF in renal and respiratory failure

The most serious cases of acute renal failure are usually associated with respiratory failure due to adult respiratory distress syndrome (ARDS). The use of positive end expiratory pressure ventilation and strategies to dry lungs out are standard practice.

Haemofiltration has been used successfully in ARDS without renal failure and claims have been made that benefits result from the filtering of vasoactive peptides[13].

Haemofiltration can achieve dehydration without cardiovascular upset and deal with the hypercatabolic patient. Figure 2.10 illustrates a case of acute renal failure complicated by ARDS (Apache II[4] score on admission = 21) in which the dominant therapy was haemofiltration consisting of 18–24 L fluid exchanges and blood flow rates of 300–400 ml/min via a radial Scribner shunt. Treatment times were between 2.5 and 4 hours. Haemofiltration was undertaken on 38 occasions, haemodialysis (using PPF primed dialysers) on 11 occasions (3-4 hours for comparative purposes). The biochemical changes were similar in both treatment regimes as shown in Table 2.3.

The differences between haemodialysis, CAVH and haemofiltration in relation to the management of patients with acute renal failure are shown in Table 2.4.

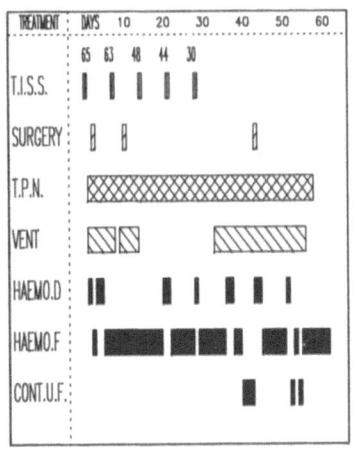
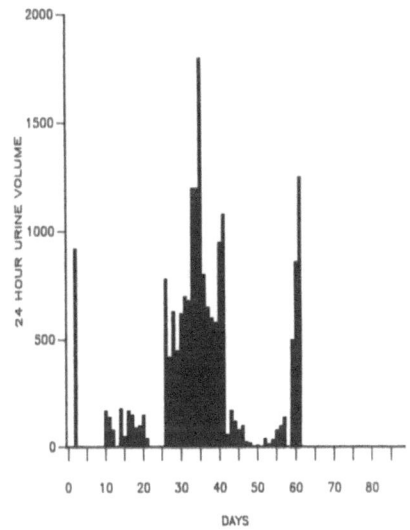

FIGURE 2.10 Acute renal and respiratory failure secondary to biliary peritonitis and bronchopneumonia (TISS[15])

TABLE 2.3   Biochemical changes following HD (3 h) and HF (24 L/4 h)

HD				HF			
Urea (mmol/L)		Creatinine (μmol/L)		Urea (mmol/L)		Creatinine (μmol/L)	
Pre	Post	Pre	Post	Pre	Post	Pre	Post
67	36	390	295	44	32	440	320
46	32	460	335	40	27	455	315
39	33	415	370	38.5	24	375	255
28.5	19.5	355	275	28.5	17.5	345	255
28	20	395	325	24	15	350	225
29	18	320	220	22.5	15	310	230
41	27	505	350	37.5	28	390	270

HAEMOFILTRATION IN PATIENTS WITH END-STAGE RENAL DISEASE

The high cost of haemofiltration has prevented it overtaking haemo-dialysis as the mainstay of therapy for patients with chronic renal failure. Its benefits, however, make it the treatment of choice for certain types of patients and those with particular problems associated with conventional haemodialysis.

Treatment – associated disorders

Hypotension, accompanied by muscle cramps, nausea and vomiting, has been reported as a complication of haemodialysis in 10–25% treatment sessions[16], especially in vulnerable patients – the elderly, those with pre-existing cardiac disease and those with autonomic neuropathy, e.g. diabetic patients. These symptoms are more common when excess weight gain between dialyses makes removal of large

TABLE 2.4   Comparative features of HD, HF and CAVH in acute renal failure

	Advantages	Disadvantages
HD	1. Inexpensive 2. Efficient biochemical control 3. Suitable for hyperkalaemic and hypercatabolic patients	1. Cardiovascular instability 2. PPF prime often required 3. Dialysis plumbing required 4. Variable acid–base homeostasis 5. Hypoxaemia 6. Intermittent ultrafiltration
HF	1. Cardiovascular stability 2. Ultrafiltration potential greater than HD 3. Suitable for hyperkalaemic and hypercatabolic patients 4. Automated	1. High blood flow rate required (15 gauge minimum cannula size) 2. Intermittent ultrafiltration 3. Expensive
CAVH	1. Simple, inexpensive 2. Continuous ultrafiltration facilitates nutrition 3. Cardiovascular stability	1. Ineffective in patients who are hypercatabolic, have large haematoma, gross haemolysis, rhabdomyolysis or hyperkalaemia 2. Continuous anticoagulation 3. Femoral cannulation 4. Prolonged patient immobilization 5. Fluid balancing problems 6. Nurse intensive 7. Drug removal[9]

quantities of fluid necessary during a treatment session. Haemofiltration has been shown significantly to reduce the incidence of hypotension and cramps when patients were treated with both modalities[17] (Table 2.5). These findings have been confirmed in many

49

TABLE 2.5   Complications of haemofiltration and haemodialysis

Complication	Haemofiltration (n=33112)		Haemodialysis (n=41510)	
	Number	%	Number	%
Muscle cramps	1125	3.4	2360	5.7
Hypotensive reactions	1035	3.1	4152	10.0
Hypertensive reactions	950	2.9	1270	3.1
Fever reactions	84	0.3	112	0.3
Fluid removal (ml/h)	680	±210	395	±122

Reproduced with kind permission from Quellhorst, E. A. (1986). Long-term survival. In Henderson, L. W. et al. (eds.) Haemofiltration, p. 224, Springer-Verlag.

other studies despite more rapid removal of fluid in the haemofiltration treatments[18]. Patients with cardiac disease have reduced treatment-associated hypotension, angina and cramps with haemofiltration, whereas modifications of conventional dialysis, such as sequential ultrafiltration and bicarbonate dialysis have made only a marginal difference[16]. No difference in the incidence of ventricular arrhythmias has been found between haemofiltration and haemodialysis in patients with pre-existing cardiac disease[19]. Blood pressure is higher after haemofiltration than after haemodialysis. The increased stability of the cardiovascular system seems to be due to the maintenance (and sometimes increase) in peripheral resistance during haemofiltration, whereas, in haemodialysis, peripheral resistance falls[20]. Catecholamine levels are maintained and levels rise with ultrafiltration, whereas, in conventional haemodialysis, levels fall with fluid removal. Extracellular fluid volume is reduced to a lesser extent with haemofiltration as more fluid shifts from intracellular to extracellular compartments[21]. These changes are not mediated by changes in baroreceptor function or body temperature[22]. Retention of plasma proteins during ultrafiltration increases osmotic pressure and leads to a plasma refilling rate of 65% of the fluid lost by ultrafiltration, whereas this is as low as 40%

in haemodialysis[23]. This difference may account for the maintenance of peripheral resistance and the lower incidence of hypotension in patients treated with haemofiltration.

Control of hypertension

Hypertension in patients with end-stage renal disease is due to excess salt and water retention in about 90% of cases. Adequate fluid removal will control blood pressure in these patients. In the remaining 10%, hypertension is volume independent, usually associated with elevated levels of plasma renin due to loss of the normal inverse relationship between exchangeable sodium and plasma renin activity. This latter group does not respond to fluid removal by lowering blood pressure[23]. Haemofiltration may benefit those with volume-dependent hypertension, especially where dialysis-associated hypotension and associated symptoms prevent adequate fluid removal with haemodialysis. Haemofiltration enables a progressive reduction in weight without side effects and patients generally tolerate higher volumes of fluid removal with haemofiltration than with haemodialysis[20,23].

Renal osteodystrophy

Calcium balance in haemofiltration depends on the amount of calcium in the substitution fluid, fluid balance – as removal of a large amount of fluid may lead to negative calcium balance, and the plasma concentration of ionized calcium[24]. Calcium balance can thus be controlled by adjustments in the calcium concentration of the substitution fluid in order to prevent calcium loss. Phosphate elimination occurs during the first half of the treatment[24]. There is a delayed rebound in plasma phosphate level after haemofiltration suggesting slowed diffusion of the bound form between cellular and extracellular compartments[25,26]. Haemofiltration achieves satisfactory phosphate removal with reduced need for oral phosphate binding agents such as calcium carbonate and aluminium hydroxide[27]. Conflicting data on plasma parathyroid hormone concentrations has been obtained in haemofiltration[21,27]. The discrepancy in findings may be explained by differences in calcium balance. No change in renal osteodystrophy as determined by bone X-rays and densitometry was found when patients were changed from haemodialysis to haemofiltration. No difference in the incidence and severity of osteitis fibrosa was found when bone biopsies from haemodialysis and haemofiltration patients were compared after two years of treatment[29]; no aluminium osteomalacia was found. Aluminium and iron removal after desferrioxamine infusion was higher with haemofiltration[30]. Plasma concentrations of 25-(OH)D were decreased in patients receiving haemofiltration, possibly because of losses in the filtrate; plasma levels should be monitored to allow appropriate supplementation to be started as necessary[29,36].

Metabolic effects

Removal of urea and creatinine is less effective with haemofiltration than with haemodialysis. Slight elevations of blood urea and creatinine concentrations occur when patients are transferred from haemodialysis to haemofiltration. These, however, stabilize at new levels. Uraemic complications, such as pericarditis, pleuritis and progressive neuropathy, are seldom seen, and, when already present, rarely progress after patients transfer from haemodialysis to haemofiltration[27]. Haemofiltration is more efficient than haemodialysis in removing molecules of higher molecular weight (15 000–50 000 daltons)[27] and there are many more reports linking uraemic complications with these larger molecules. The improved clearance of these substances may account for apparent clinical improvement.

Alterations in various hormone levels also occur in haemofiltration. Many of these substances fall to within the appropriate molecular weight range and are removed in the ultrafiltrate. Reduction in levels of growth hormone, thyroid stimulating hormone, thyroxine and triiodothyronine all occur, but there is no evidence of hypothyroidism developing as the T4/TBG ratio remains stable[31,32]. There is a significant increase in the plasma bicarbonate concentration in haemofiltration patients, both acutely and long term. Blood pH is also higher than in patients receiving standard acetate haemodialysis. No significant differences in pO_2 and pCO_2 occur during haemofiltration compared with haemodialysis treatment[33], cholesterol levels are not better with haemofiltration than with haemodialysis, and there is no improvement in lipid profiles.

Haemofiltration removes substantial amounts of β_2-microglobulin (molecular weight 11 600 Da), about 80% of daily production[34,35]. This substance has been implicated in the development of carpal tunnel syndrome in long-term haemodialysis patients due to dialysis-associated amyloid deposition but it remains to be seen whether haemofiltration is capable of preventing this complication.

Haemofiltration in children

Haemofiltration has been reported as being used successfully in children with end-stage renal disease[28,31]. Twenty-three children, aged 2 years and upwards, were haemofiltered[28] using Cimino fistulae, bovine grafts, Scribner shunts and subclavian vein catheters with a mean blood flow of 224 ml/min. Blood pressure was stable during haemofiltration when compared with haemodialysis sessions in the same chronic renal failure patients and there was good cardiovascular tolerance to fluid removal in children with overhydration. Clinical side effects were recorded in 22% of the children compared with 27% during haemodialysis. In another study, haemofiltration was also found to be better tolerated than haemodialysis, with reduction in hypotensive episodes and in dialysis-associated symptoms. Solute removal was not significantly different and treatment times were shorter. The need for high blood flows makes haemofiltration difficult in very small children although CAVH has been used successfully in small infants with refractory cardiac failure[36] and with multiple organ system failure[37].

Long-term results of haemofiltration

As well as fewer side effects, there are other long-term advantages of haemofiltration. Hospitalization rates are lower with haemofiltration than with haemodialysis or CAPD[18]. Infection is the single most common reason for admission in all groups; hypotension, hyper-

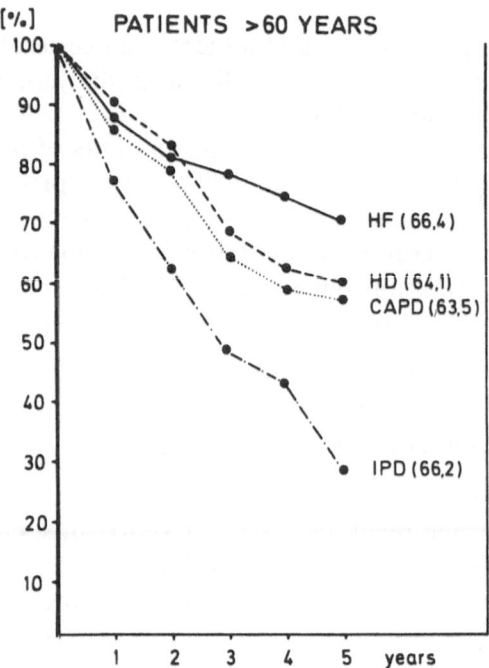

HAEMODIALYSIS

[%] PATIENTS >60 YEARS

HF (66,4)

HD (64,1)
CAPD (63,5)

IPD (66,2)

FIGURE 2.11 Survival rates of patients older than 60 years of age with end-stage renal failure depending on treatment modalities; mean age in parentheses (reproduced by kind permission from Quellhorst, E. A. (1986). Long-term survival. In Henderson, L. W. *et al.* (eds.) *Haemofiltration*, p. 229, Springer-Verlag)

tension and cerebrovascular disease are frequently encountered in the haemodialysis group, while vascular access problems, together with malignancies and myocardial infarction, predominate in the haemofiltration patients[18]. Overall survival rates for low-risk patients are no different with haemodialysis or with haemofiltration, but, for high-risk patients, benefits of haemofiltration are evident. Elderly renal patients treated with haemofiltration show better survival at any chosen time interval than those treated with acetate dialysis[38,39] (Figure 2.11).

Diabetic patients also have lower hospitalization rates on haemofiltration and survival rates comparable with CAPD have been reported[39] (Figure 2.12). Hypertension and myocardial insufficiency were also treated more effectively by haemofiltration than haemo-

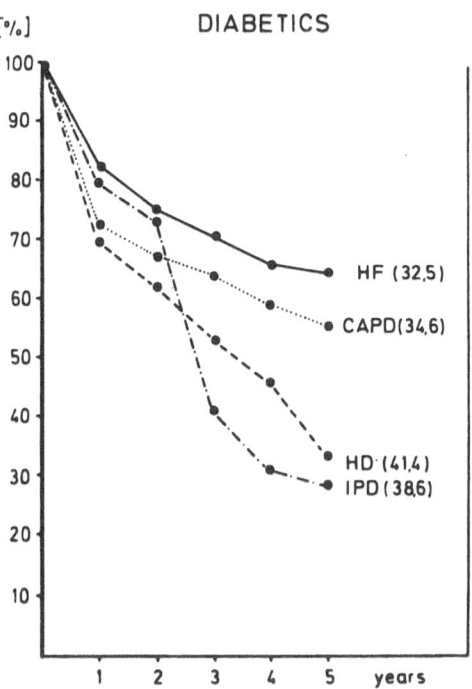

FIGURE 2.12 Survival rates of patients with diabetic nephropathy depending on treatment modalities (reproduced by kind permission from Quellhorst, E. A. (1986). Long-term survival. In Henderson, L. W. *et al.* (eds.) *Haemofiltration*, p. 231, Springer-Verlag)

dialysis. Diabetic complications, such as retinopathy and neuropathy were, however, reported more frequently with haemofiltration than with CAPD[18]. Thus, CAPD is the treatment of choice for patients with diabetes mellitus in end-stage renal failure.

Complications of treatment

Infusion of large volumes of ready-prepared substitution fluid during each treatment carries the risks of introducing pathogens and pyrogens into the blood stream. Febrile reactions occur in 0.19% of treatments (1 per 531)[31], and 10% of these are of sufficient severity to cause circulatory shock. It has been suggested that on-site preparation of substitution fluid, or use of a bacterial filter, may reduce the incidence of this complication[40]. As high blood flow rates (greater than 200 ml/min) are needed, adequate vascular access is necessary. Problems relating to the A-V fistulae are a common reason for admission to hospital for patients on haemofiltration and inadequate vascular access remains the main reason for treatment failure[18].

Quantitation and prescription of haemofiltration

At present, guide lines for adequate haemofiltration therapy are not well developed. The amount of treatment is determined as litres of plasma water exchanged per treatment (or per week). Adjustment for patient size is made and prescription may be for 1/3 of body weight per treatment or 40–45% of body weight per session[17]. These rough calculations make no allowances for differing nutritional needs or differing haemofilters[41]. A simple approach allows for differences in dietary protein intake using the formula:

$$\text{Ultrafiltrate} = \frac{\text{DPI} \times 0.12 \times 7}{0.70}$$

where ultrafiltrate is number of litres exchanged per week and DPI is daily protein intake in grams[42].

Haemofiltration will never completely replace haemodialysis as long as it remains so much more expensive. It is, however, indicated for those patients who suffer from severe dialysis-related hypotension, cramps, nausea and vomiting. Patients with cardiovascular instability, especially those with cardiac disease, autonomic dysfunction and the elderly who may not tolerate fluid removal on haemodialysis, should be considered for haemofiltration as should those diabetic patients for whom CAPD is not possible[21]. Advances in the production of substitution fluid and re-use of filters may reduce costs and allow haemofiltration to be undertaken more widely for patients with ESRD[39].

ACKNOWLEDGEMENTS

Acknowledgements are due to Sister J. K. Gibbins and Renal Nursing Services whose skills make advances in therapy possible and to our renal secretaries, Mrs C. Watson and Miss J. Cook, for their tolerance.

REFERENCES

1. Eisenhauer Th. (1985). Continuous arteriovenous haemofiltration (CAVH). In Sieberth H. G. and Mann H. (Eds.) *Conference on continuous arteriovenous hemofiltration (CAVH)*, Aachen (FRG) Karger Basel 1–13
2. Henderson L., Besarb A., Michaels A. and Bluemle L. W. (1967). Blood purification by ultrafiltration and fluid replacement (dialfiltration). *Trans. Am. Soc. Artif. Intern. Organs*, **16,** 216–222
3. Okazaki M. and Yoshida F. (1976). Ultrafiltration of blood: Effect of hematocrit on ultrafiltration rate. *Ann. Biomed. Eng.*, **4,** 138
4. Silverstein M. E., Ford C. A., Lysaght M. J. and Henderson L. W. (1974). The treatment of intractable fluid overload. *N. Engl. J. Med.*, **291,** 747
5. Teschan, P. E., Baxter, C. R., O'Brien, T. F., Freyhof, J. N. and Hall, W. H. (1960). Prophylactic haemodialysis in the treatment of acute renal failure. *Ann. Intern. Med.*, **53,** 992
6. Kleinknech, D., Jungers, P., Chanard, J., Barbanel, C., Ganeval, D. and Rondon-Nucete, M. (1971). Factors influencing immediate prognosis in acute renal failure with special reference to prophylactic haemodialysis. *Adv. Nephrol.*, **1,** 207–230
7. Easterling, R. E. and Forland, M. (1964). A five year experience with prophylactic dialysis for acute renal failure. *Trans. Am. Soc. Artif. Intern. Organs*, **10,** 200–206
8. Olbricht, C. J., Schurek, H. J., Stolte, H. and Koch, K. M. (1985). The influence of vascular access mode on the efficiency of CAVH in continuous arterio-venous hemofiltration (CAVH). In Sieberth, H. G. and Mann, H. (eds.) *International Conference on CAVH*, Aschen, Karger, Basel, pp. 14–24
9. Golper, T. A. (1985). Continuous arteriovenous hemofiltration in acute renal failure. *Am. J. Kidney Dis.*, **6,** 373–386
10. Kohen, J. A., Whitley, K. Y. and Kjellstrand, C. M. (1985). Continuous arteriovenous hemofiltration: A comparison with hemodialysis in acute renal failure. *Trans. Am. Soc. Artif. Intern. Organs*, **31,** 169–175
11. Baldamus, C. A. (1986). Hemodynamics in hemofiltration. In Henderson, L. W., Quellhorst, E. A., Baldamus, C. A. and Lysaght, M. J. (eds.) *Hemofiltration*, pp. 155–200. (Berlin, Heidelberg, New York, Tokyo: Springer–Verlag)
12. Bosch, J. P. and Laner, A. (1986). Acid–base balance in hemofiltration. In Henderson, L. W., Quellhorst, E. A., Baldamus, C. A. and Lysaght, M. J. (eds.) *Hemofiltration*, pp. 147–154. (Berlin, Heidelberg, New York, Toyko: Springer–Verlag)
13. Gotloib, L., Barzilay, E., Shustak, A., Wais, Z., Jaichenko, J. and Lev, A. (1986). Hemofiltration in septic ARDS. The artificial kidney as an artificial endocrine lung. *Resuscitation*, **13,** 123–132

14. Knaus, W. A., Zimmerman, J. E., Wagner, D. P., Draper, E. A. and Lawrence, D. E. (1981). APACHE – acute physiology and chronic health evaluation: a physiologically based classification system. *Crit. Care Med.*, **9**, 591–597
15. Keene, A. R. and Cullen, D. J. (1983). Therapeutic intervention scoring system: update 1983. *Crit. Care Med.*, **11**, 1–3
16. Davison, A. M., Roberts, T. G., Mascie-Taylor, B. H. and Lewins, A. M. (1982). Haemofiltration for profound dialysis-induced hypotension: removal of sodium and water without blood-pressure change. *Br. Med. J.*, **285**, 87–89
17. Baldamus Conrad, A. (1983) Clinical value and technical feasibility of long-term haemofiltration. *ASAIO J.*, **6, 4**, 192–196
18. Quellhorst, E. A., Schuenemann, B. and Hildebrand, U. (1983). Morbidity and mortality in long-term haemofiltration. *ASAIO J.*, **6**, 185–191
19. Wizemann, V., Kramer, W., Funke, T. and Schutterle, G. (1985). Dialysis-induced cardiac arrythmias: fact or fiction? *Nephron*, **39**, 356–360
20. Henderson Lee, W. (1987). Hemofiltration. *Kidney*, **20**, 6, 25–30
21. Glabman, S. and Lauer, A. (1986). Selection of patients for haemofiltration. In Henderson *et al.* (eds.) *Haemofiltration*, pp. 115–118. (Berlin, Heidelberg, New York, Tokyo: Springer–Verlag)
22. Henderson Lee, W. (1986). Heterogeneity of the cardiovascular response to haemofiltration. *Kidney Int.*, **29**, 901–907
23. Quellhorst, E. A. (1986). Blood pressure control. In Henderson *et al.* (eds.) *Haemofiltration*, pp. 201–210. (Berlin, Heidelberg, New York, Tokyo: Springer–Verlag)
24. Schneider, H. (1982). Electrolyte balance during haemofiltration treatment. *Contr. Nephrol.*, **32**, 111–118
25. Haas, T., Dongradi, G., Villeboeuf, F., De Viel, E., Fournier, J. F. and Duruy, D. (1983). Plasma kinetics of small molecules during and after haemofiltration: Decrease in haemofiltration efficiency related to increase in ultrafiltration rate. *Clin. Nephrol.*, **19**, 193–200
26. Pogglitsch, H., Petek, W., Ziak, E., Sterz, F. and Holzer, H. (1984). Phosphorus kinetics during haemodialysis and haemofiltration. *Proc. EDTA-ERA*, **21**, 461–467
27. Schaefer, K. and Von Herrath, D. (1986). Impact of haemofiltration on various metabolic and endocrine disturbances of chronic uraemia. In Henderson *et al.* (eds.) *Haemofiltration*, pp. 211–220. (Berlin, Heidelberg, New York, Tokyo: Springer–Verlag)
28. Muller-Wiefel, D. E., Rauh, W., Wingen, A. M., Mehls, O. and Scharer, K. (1982). Haemofiltration in children. *Contr. Nephrol.*, **32**, 128–136
29. Sebert, J. L., Fournier, A., Leflon, P., Fohrer, P., de Fremont, J. F., Moriniere, Ph., Galy, Cl., Marie, A., Demonts, R., Boudailliez, B., Gueris, J., Dkhissi, H., Garabedian, M. and Lambrey, G. (1986). Comparative evaluation of bone aluminium content and bone histology in patients on chronic haemodialysis and haemofiltration. *Nephron.*, **42**, 34–40
30. Baldamus, C. A., Schmidt, H., Scheuermann, E. H., Werner, E., Kaltwasser, J. P. and Schoeppe, W. (1984). Desferrioxamine treatment for aluminium and iron overload in uraemic patients treated by haemodialysis or haemofiltration. *Proc. EDTA-ERA*, **21**, 382–386
31. Pascual, J. F., Lopes, J. D. and Molina, M. (1987). Hemofiltration in children with renal failure. *Paediatr. Clin. N. Am.*, **34**, 3, 803–817

32. Locsey, L., Lenhey, A. and Leovey, A. (1987). Hormonal changes in haemo-dialysed and in kidney transplanted patients. *Int. Urol. Nephrol. (Hungary)*, **19** (2), 201–213
33. Bosch, J. P. and Lauer, A. (1986). Acid-based balance in haemofiltration. In Henderson *et al.* (eds.) *Haemofiltration*, pp. 147–154. (Berlin, Heidelberg, New York, Tokyo: Springer–Verlag)
34. Kaiser, J. P., Hagemann, J., von Herrath, D. and Schaefer, K. (1988). Different handling of beta$_2$-microglobulin during haemodialysis and haemofiltration. *Nephron*, **48**, 132–135
35. Floge, J., Granolleras, C., Bingel, M., Deschodt, G., Branger, B., Oules, R., Koch, K. M. and Shaldon, S. (1987). Beta$_2$-microglobulin kinetics in haemodialysis and haemofiltration. *Nephrol. Dial. Transplant*, 1 (4), 223–228
36. Zobel, G., Beitzke, A., Stein, J. I. and Trop, M. (1987). Continuous arteriovenous haemofiltration in children with post-operative cardiac failure. *Br. Heart J.*, **58** (5), 473–476
37. Zobel, G., Trop, M., Ring, E. and Grubbauer, H. M. (1987). Arteriovenous hemofiltration in children with multiple organ system failure. *Int. J. Artif. Organs (Italy)*, **10** (4), 233–238
38. Schaefer, K., Asmus, G., Quellhorst, E., Pauls, A., von Herrath, D. and Jahnke, J. (1984). Optimum dialysis treatment for patients over 60 years with primary renal disease. Survival data and clinical results from 242 patients treated either by haemodialysis or haemofiltration. *Proc. EDTA-ERA*, **21**, 510–517
39. Quellhorst, E. A. (1986). Long-term survival. In Henderson *et al.* (eds.) *Haemo-filtration*, pp. 221–232. (Berlin, Heidelberg, New York, Tokyo: Springer–Verlag)
40. Keshaviah, P. and Leuhmann, D. (1984). The importance of water treatment in haemodialysis and haemofiltration. *Proc. EDTA-ERA*, **21**, 111–129
41. Henderson, L. W. and Leypoldt, J. K. (1986). Quantitation and prescription of therapy. In Henderson *et al.* (eds.) *Haemofiltration*, pp. 129–145. (Berlin, Heidelberg, New York, Tokyo: Springer–Verlag)
42. Bosch, J. P., von Albertini, B. and Glabmans, S. (1982). Prescription for haemo-filtration. *Contr. Nephrol.*, **31**, 137–145

3

CLINICAL HAEMOPERFUSION

J. F. WINCHESTER

Haemoperfusion, the direct contact of blood with sorbents within cartridges, has been used as an adjunct to dialysis for uraemia, and in drug intoxication, hepatic encephalopathy and for a variety of other conditions which will be outlined.

PRINCIPLES OF HAEMOPERFUSION

Available haemoperfusion devices consist of plastic chambers with particulate sorbent materials within them, through which blood percolates. Bioincompatibility of early haemoperfusion systems[1,2] was improved by microencapsulation of the sorbent particles within a polymer membrane[3] such as collodion (cellulose nitrate). The haemoperfusion device with inlet and outlet blood lines for connection to vascular access, a blood pump, gauges to detect pressure drops across the column, indicating clotting within the device, and intermittent or continuous use of herapin or prostacyclin to prevent blood coagulation within the extracorporeal circulation is the basic requirement for the procedure. Typical sorbents used in haemoperfusion devices are activated carbons (charcoals), ion-exchange resins or non-ionic macroporous resins. All devices now available use coated activated charcoal, either as granular charcoal coated with cellulose nitrate (Chang's model), or with acrylic hydrogel polymer, or heparinized copolymer. Other devices containing charcoals are prepared from extruded charcoal, coated with either cellulose acetate or methacrylic hydrogel, or consist of columns containing spherical petroleum-based charcoal coated with cellulose nitrate. Non-ionic resins, consisting of macroporous cross-linked polystyrene amberlite series, such as XAD-2 and XAD-4, are also available.

The devices used in clinical studies commonly contain 70–300 g activated charcoal coated with polymer membranes ranging in thickness from 0.05–0.5 μm. The devices are described below and in Table 3.1.

Solutes adsorbed

The uraemic solutes adsorbed are shown in Table 3.2 and range in molecular mass from 60 to 21 500 daltons depending on the polymer membrane thickness. Substantial reduction in the adsorption of higher molecular weight substances (more than 3500 Da) occurs with polymer coating[4] but smaller molecules are little affected. It is the capacity to adsorb molecules of the 'middle molecular weight' size (300–1500 Da) that has stimulated interest in activated charcoal haemoperfusion in uraemia. Glucose, calcium, amino acids, hormones, middle molecules and trace metals, such as arsenic, cobalt, chromium and selenium are all adsorbed[5].

TABLE 3.1   Available haemoperfusion devices

Manufacturer	Device	Sorbent type	Amount of sorbent	Polymer coating
Erika	Hemocart or Alukart	Petroleum-based charcoal	60 or 155 g	Collodion
Gambro	Adsorba	Norit	100 or 300 g	Cellulose acetate
Smith and Nephew	Haemocol	Sutcliffe Speakman charcoal	100 or 300 g	Acrylic hydrogel
Extracorporeal* or Braun	XR-004	XAD-4 resin	350 g	None

* = no longer available in USA

TABLE 3.2   Uraemic toxins removed by sorbents

Adrenocorticotrophin	Middle molecule peaks
(Aldosterone)	Myoinositol
Amino acids	Non-protein nitrogen
Calcium	Nor-epinephrine
25,OH-Cholecalciferol	Organic acids
Creatinine	Oxalate
Cyclic AMP	Parathyroid hormone
Epinephrine	Phenols
Folic acid	(Phosphate)
Fibronectin	Polyamino acids
Gastrin	(Renin)
Glucagon	Ribonuclease
Glucose	Serotonin
(Growth hormone)	Thyroxine
Guanidines	Trace metals: As, Co, Cr, Se
Indoles	Triglycerides
Insulin	Triiodothyronine
L-dopamine	(Urea)
Lysozyme	Uric acid
(Magnesium)	Vitamin B_{12}

() poorly removed

Side effects of haemoperfusion

Particle embolization, a feature of early devices, has been improved
by selecting charcoal resistant to attrition, developing polymer coating
techniques and applying washing procedures on a commercial scale.
Platelet depletion observed with early uncoated charcoal haemoperfusion devices[1,2,6] has largely been overcome with the introduction
of microencapsulation techniques; in uraemia, current haemoperfusion devices produce platelet losses of 30% or less[7]. Chang's
coating technique[3,8] and hydrophilic methacrylate-coated charcoal[9]
are particularly haemocompatible (Table 3.2). Transient leukopaenia,
similar to that noted during haemodialysis, occurs during haemoperfusion. Minor reductions in plasma fibrinogen[1,2] and fibronectin[10]
concentrations have been observed in uraemic patients even with
polymer-coated activated charcoal devices[11]; no appreciable changes
in coagulation factors II–XII have, however, been noted[11]. The

haemostatic changes may be particularly profound in patients with hepatic failure and have led to the use of prostacyclin for anti-coagulation during haemoperfusion of patients in hepatic coma[12].

Other side effects of haemoperfusion, such as removal of calcium or glucose, are easily overcome, as is the small reduction in body temperature (no blood warming devices are incorporated in the apparatus). Pyrogenic reactions observed with the early charcoal haemo-perfusion devices[1] are rarely seen with modern devices. Hormones and trace metals are also adsorbed by activated charcoal devices[5,9,11].

HAEMOPERFUSION IN URAEMIA

In 1948, Muirhead and Reid[13] used ion exchange resins (amberlite IR-100 H and deacidite) contained in a haemoperfusion device to remove urea but severe side effects (pyrogenic reactions, electrolyte disturbances and haemolysis) precluded further use of this resin. In 1964, Yatzidis[1] reported that uncoated activated charcoal haemoperfusion could adsorb *in vitro* 2 g of barbital, phenobarbital and pentobarbital and 2.6 g of salicylic acid and glutethimide. Extension of the work to uraemic patients[1] demonstrated that creatinine, uric acid, guanidine, indoles, phenolic compounds and organic acids could be removed. In 1965, Yatzidis *et al.*[14] used activated uncoated carbon haemoperfusion to treat successfully two patients with barbiturate poisoning. Since then, many studies have confirmed these observations and improved the side-effect profile. Chang *et al.*[15] confirmed that, in uraemic man, charcoal haemoperfusion could remove uraemic toxins, including polyamino acids and medium molecular weight substances[16,17] (Table 3.2). These reports, and many others, have shown, however, that urea could not be adsorbed in the quantities thought necessary for the treatment of uraemia. Some of the long-term studies of haemo-perfusion in uremia are outlined in detail in Table 3.3

Most short-term studies have not reported any clinical improvement with the use of charcoal haemoperfusion in uremia. However, improvement in pericarditis[1,18], gastrointestinal symptoms[1] and leth-argy[1], as well as cardiac function[19], have been observed.

Charcoal haemoperfusion alone is insufficient to control the symptoms of uraemia, or remove water from uraemic subjects (Table 3.2)

TABLE 3.3 Clinical studies of haemoperfusion in uraemia

First author (reference)	Duration of study	(Hours/wk)	Number of subjects	Sorbent system and methods	Solute removed (clearance (ml/min) or % fall in plasma level)	Adverse effects and comments
Stefoni (20)	1–12 months 1 or 2 HP/HD/week	3–5	18	Hydroxy-methacrylate-coated Norit charcoal, initially 300 g then 150 g with HD	HP Cr (77), UA (55) Vitamin B$_{12}$ (31) HP/HD Cr (174), UA (119)	Platelets unchanged hypotension, cramps, headache, pyrexia, improved neuropathy and well being
Bonomini (24)	1–36 months (mean 7.5 months) 2 HP/HD/week	8–10	27	Hydroxy-methacrylate-coated Norit charcoal, 150 g with HD	Water retention (9/27) solute clearances as in above	Stable MNCV other side effects as in above
Henderson (23)	10 months 3 HP/HD/week (controls 3 HD)	15	9	Sutcliffe Speakman acrylic hydrogel coated charcoal 100 g HP with HD	—	Improved wellbeing
Chang (22)	6 month crossover with 12 h HD/week	8	4	ACAC DiaKart petroleum based 70 g with HD	—	No change in biochemistry, haematology, etc.
Barre (25)	4–6 months 2 or 3 HD/HP/week	8	5	ACAC DiaKart petroleum based 70 g with HD	—	No increased heparin requirement, cost effective, improved pericarditis, neuropathy, hypercaogulability

Abbreviations: ACAC = albumin collodion (= cellulose nitrate) coated charcoal; HP = haemoperfusion; HD = haemodialysis; Cr = creatinine; UA = uric acid; Ca = calcium; MMS = middle molecular weight substances; MNCV = mean nerve conduction velocity

In long-term studies, therefore, charcoal haemoperfusion must be combined with haemodialysis or ultrafiltration devices. Improvements in mean nerve conduction velocity[20,21], electromyogram, pruritis and pericarditis[21], and reduction in dialysis time[20,22] have been observed by some, but not by all, investigators. Changes in nerve conduction velocity, for example, were not seen in the study by Henderson and Kennedy[23]. Adverse reactions are frequent and include hypotension[20], flushing, fever, chills, nausea and headaches[20,24] and an inability to maintain fluid balance in some[20,24], but not all[22,23] patients.

A reduction in blood urea concentration was observed by Stefoni *et al.*[20] but not by others[22,23]. Combined haemoperfusion/ haemodialysis has been calculated to add 30% to the annual cost of dialysis[20] but Barre *et al.*[25] found the addition of haemoperfusion to haemodialysis to be cost-effective. Solute clearances with combined haemoperfusion/haemodialysis at blood flow rates of 200 ml/min are as follows: urea 143–160 ml/min, creatinine 168–174 ml/min, urate 119–194 ml/min, and 'middle molecules' 51–165 ml/min.

The wide spectrum of adsorptive qualities possessed by charcoal and the improvements in uraemic symptoms suggest that haemoperfusion may have a role in the treatment of uraemia. As urea, water, electrolytes and hydrogen ions are not removed, it is necessary to combine haemosorbent removal of solutes with dialysis or ultrafiltration. In the future, sorbents will probably be used in a hybrid device which will combine all the properties currently achieved by haemodialysis but with greater efficiency. The devices available at present are biocompatible for repetitive use but the cost of haemoperfusion has limited its widespread acceptance. Haemoperfusion devices range in cost from £60–200 and are too expensive for long-term use. If costs were to approximate those for conventional haemodialysers, haemoperfusion might be used more widely. At present, it seems justifiable to use these high-cost devices in the treatment of specific dialysis problems, i.e. treatment of aluminium and iron overload syndromes, peripheral neuropathy and pericarditis.

TABLE 3.4   Drugs and chemicals removed with haemoperfusion

Barbiturates
Amobarbital
Butabarbital
Hexabarbital
Pentobarbital
Phenobarbital
Quinalbital
Secobarbital
Thiopental
Vinalbital

**Non-barbiturate
hypnotics,
sedatives,
tranquilizers**
Carbromal
Chloral hydrate
Chlorpromazine
(Diazepam)
Diphenhydramine
Ethchlorvynol
Glutethimide
Meprobamate
Methaqualone
Methsuximide
Methyprylon
Promazine
Promethazine

**Analgesics,
antirheumatic**
Acetaminophen
Acetylsalicylic acid
Colchicine
d-Propoxyphene
Methylsalicylate
Phenylbutazone
Salicylic acid

**Antimicrobials/
anticancer**
(Adriamycin)
Ampicillin
Carmustine
Chloramphenicol
Chloroquine
Clindamycin
Dapsone
Doxorubicin
Gentamicin
Isoniazid
(Methotrexate)
Thiabendazole

Antidepressants
Amitryptiline)
(Imipramine)
(Tricyclics)

**Plants, animals,
herbicides,
insecticides**
Amanitin
Chlordane
Demeton sulfoxide
Dimethoate
Diquat
Methylparathion
Nitrostigmine
Organophosphates
Phalloidin
Polychlorinated
  biphenyls
Paraquat
Parathion

Cardiovascular
Digoxin
Diltiazem
(Disopyramide)
Metoprolol
n-Acetylprocainamide
Procainamide
Quinidine
(Aluminium)*
(Iron)*

Miscellaneous
Aminophylline
Cimetidine
(Fluoroacetamide)
(Phencyclidine)
Phenols
(Podophyllin)
Theophylline

Solvents, gases
Carbon tetrachloride
Ethylene oxide
Trichloroethanol

() not well removed; ()* removed with chelating agent

DRUG INTOXICATION

A large number of patients present as medical emergencies to hospitals as a result of acute self-poisoning; about 5% of those admitted require treatment to eliminate poisons[26]. About 85% of cases referred to US Poison Control Centers can be managed by telephone consultation and follow up[27]. In the United Kingdom, over the 10-year period up to 1984, there were 38 024 poisoning deaths[28]. In the United States, it is estimated that, for 1985, there were 1.9 million poisoning incidents[29]. There were 328 deaths from poisoning reported to Poison Control Centers and haemodialysis was used in 217 cases and haemoperfusion in 56[29].

Treatment should follow management guidelines[30], using intensive care without the use of central stimulants[31]. In very severely poisoned patients, dialysis for removing drugs, as well as haemoperfusion, has been adopted. This subject has been reviewed in depth[32-34]. Haemodialysis is an effective method for removing highly diffusible substances, while haemoperfusion is more efficient with regard to certain other poisons. Lipid-soluble drugs and protein-bound drugs, which are inefficiently removed by haemodialysis, can be removed more efficiently by haemoperfusion.

Drugs removed by haemoperfusion are shown in Table 3.4. Most studies have dealt principally with activated charcoal haemoperfusion, less commonly with non-ionic macroporous resin haemoperfusion, and rarely with ion-exchange resin haemoperfusion. Extraction efficiency for drug removal (Table 3.5) gives guidance in choosing devices for treatment of poisoned patients. Fat-soluble drugs are most efficiently removed with the macroporous, non-ionic resin, XAD-4, while intoxication with water-soluble small molecules, especially, when acidosis is present, is more readily treated with haemodialysis, which, unlike haemoperfusion, corrects the acidosis. Activated charcoal haemoperfusion is less specific and can be used in a wide variety of clinical poisonings.

Using pharmacokinetic modelling, it can be demonstrated that drug elimination may be substantially enhanced with haemoperfusion[35-37]. Adverse reactions, similar to those seen in the treatment of uraemia, are of less concern since repetitive haemoperfusion is required only rarely – in poisoning with glutethimide, ethchlorvynol or with other

TABLE 3.5   Drug extraction ratios with different devices

	Standard haemo-dialysis	Coated or uncoated charcoal haemoperfusion	XAD-2 or XAD-4 resin haemoperfusion
Amobarbital	0.26	0.3	0.9
Acetylsalicylic acid	0.5	0.5	—
Digoxin	0.2	0.3–0.6	0.4
Glutethimide	0.16	0.65	0.8
Paracetamol	0.4	0.5	0.7
Paraquat	0.5	0.6	—
Phenobarbital	0.27	0.5	0.85
Theophylline	0.5	0.7	0.75

Calculated for blood flow rate 200 ml/min

TABLE 3.6   Clinical criteria for haemoperfusion in poisoning

1. Progressive deterioration despite intensive care.
2. Severe intoxication with mid-brain dysfunction.
3. Development of complications of coma.
4. Impairment of normal drug excretory function.
5. Intoxication with agents producing metabolic and/or delayed effects.
6. Intoxication with an extractable drug which can be removed at a greater rate than endogenous elimination.

drugs which possess slow removal rates[32]. Thrombocytopaenia developing during haemoperfusion in poisoning cases usually recovers within 24–28 h and is very rarely associated with coagulation problems[33]. Several authors argue that conservative management alone is associated with a favourable outcome[38]. There are, however, geographical and other variations in poisoning severity which must be taken into account when deciding if haemoperfusion or dialysis should be undertaken in severe cases. Small studies have suggested benefit[39], but a large-scale controlled clinical trial of haemoperfusion in poisoning has proved impossible to conduct. Clinical judgement and use of the guidelines given below is recommended when considering whether to use haemoperfusion (or haemodialysis) in poisoning.

Agents that cause metabolic abnormalities, such as acidosis, are better corrected by haemodialysis or combined haemodialysis/ haemoperfusion[40]. Haemodialysis is recommended as the treatment of choice for patients severely poisoned with ethanol, methanol, ethylene glycol and salicylate[40]. Paracetamol poisoning is best treated by administering intravenous *n*-acetylcysteine within 14 h of ingestion. Clinical trials of haemoperfusion in paracetamol poisoning have been inconclusive[41,42]. In amitriptyline poisoning, charcoal or resin haemoperfusion has been reported to be beneficial[43,44]; other investigators have not supported this view, arguing that intoxication occurs at low plasma concentrations as tricyclic drugs have large volumes of distribution[45]. Although a 60% (activated charcoal) to 90% (XAD-4 resin) extraction of nortriptyline occurs during haemoperfusion, no substantial alteration in arterial plasma drug concentrations can be detected in severe cases[45]. Haemoperfusion in digitalis poisoning has been associated with increased drug elimination rates and reduction in plasma digitalis concentrations. In renal failure patients who are at risk of digoxin intoxication, the benefits of haemoperfusion[46] might outweigh the benefits and cost of giving digitalis antibody fragments[47]. Removal of paraquat by haemoperfusion[48] has had disappointing results[49]. In severe poisoning, all therapy, including haemoperfusion[49], may not be successful, but, in certain situations, repetitive (almost continuous) activated charcoal haemoperfusion treatment can prevent pulmonary fibrosis and contribute to survival[50,51]. In theophylline poisoning, complications can be abolished with the rapid reduction of plasma theophylline concentrations with charcoal and resin haemoperfusion[52,53].

Guidelines for haemoperfusion

In addition to fulfilling clinical criteria (Table 3.6), patients should be considered for haemoperfusion only if they have also been poisoned with adsorbable drugs, such as those outlined in Table 3.4. Drug concentrations may help to determine the severity of toxicity. In mixed poisonings however, drug levels may not indicate the severity of poisoning since drug effects may be additive.

In dialysis patients, additional dialysis or haemoperfusion may be useful to remove excessive drug levels (e.g. aminoglycosides, chloramphenicol and digoxin). Digoxin intoxication is commonly encountered and may require treatment with antibodies or haemoperfusion.

Aluminium overload with bone disease (osteomalacia) or dialysis dementia has been treated with desferrioxamine in conjunction with dialysis or haemoperfusion to remove the desferrioxamine–aluminium complexes[54,55]. Clinical improvement in the renal osteodystrophy[56] and encephalopathy[57] has been reported. Iron overload in chronic dialysis patients, especially if they possess the haemochromatosis alleles (HLA A_3, B_7, B_{14})[58] has also been treated with dialysis, haemofiltration or haemoperfusion[55] in conjunction with desferrioxamine. Cardiomyopathy, diabetes and other complications may improve with such chelation treatment[59].

Heavy metals not removed efficiently by dialysis or haemoperfusion may be more efficiently removed with certain chelating agents, such as n-acetylcysteine[60] or cysteine[61]. Chelating microspheres[62] or chelate-metal groups for adsorption[61] may be useful in the future for heavy metal removal.

HAEMOPERFUSION IN HEPATIC FAILURE

Hepatic encephalopathy in fulminant hepatic failure is poorly understood. Hypotheses on pathogenesis include excessive production of mercaptans, ammonia, false neurotransmitters, altered circulating plasma branched chain:aromatic amino acid ratio and excessive production of γ-aminobutyric acid[63,64].

Chang[65] first reported improvement in consciousness in a woman treated with charcoal haemoperfusion. This report stimulated the application of charcoal haemoperfusion to the management of fulminant hepatic encephalopathy in stage IV coma. Initial studies were encouraging[18,66] but subsequent studies failed to confirm the early optimism[67]. Chang et al.[68] demonstrated that the optimum time for haemoperfusion in an experimental animal model was stage III coma.

This was subsequently confirmed in man[69], especially as the deepest coma (stage IV) was associated with a high incidence of irreversible cerebral oedema.

Studies of charcoal haemoperfusion in fulminant hepatic encephalopathy are shown in Table 3.7. In comparison with conservative therapy alone (up to 18.7% survival[70]), improved survival was achieved in some series (65% of those in stage III coma)[69]. In most series, a large number of patients recover consciousness at some point during the treatment schedule. The main goal of therapy is to induce reversal of coma for sufficiently long to allow spontaneous hepatocellular regeneration, since substances which are cytotoxic to hepatocytes *in vitro* are adsorbed on to charcoal[71]. Instituting haemoperfusion at a much earlier stage of hepatic encephalopathy is recommended.

The substances which may be relevant to the development of hepatic encephalopathy and removed by sorbent haemoperfusion are shown in Table 3.8. Recently, it has been demonstrated that serum inhibitors of brain $Na^+ K^+$ ATPase, which may play a role in the production of hepatic coma, are reduced with charcoal and resin haemoperfusion[72].

Coagulation abnormalities[73,74], associated with fulminant hepatic failure itself, may be exacerbated by haemoperfusion[75] and have caused some investigators to use prostacyclin in place of heparin as the anticoagulant for the extracorporeal circulation. The need for prostacyclin in this situation has, however, been disputed[76].

On the basis of kinetic modelling[77], haemoperfusion should be performed every 12 hours. Protein-bound substances, thought to produce hepatic coma, may not be well removed with charcoal haemoperfusion, and resin haemoperfusion[78] has been introduced.

Like uraemia, hepatic encephalopathy is probably multifactorial in origin and, at present, the design of a specific sorbent cannot be undertaken. In drug-induced liver disease[79] where the outcome is better than for hepatic failure associated with viral infections, haemoperfusion may be especially beneficial. Haemoperfusion should be used in carefully selected patients at an early stage of coma (stage III) and perhaps more frequently than previously since it probably represents the most effective available treatment for acute fulminant hepatic failure.

TABLE 3.7   Effect of haemoperfusion in fulminant hepatic encephalopathy

Study (reference)	# of patients	Recovery of consciousness	Survival	Biochemical changes and comments	Device/ anticoagulant
Gazzard et al. (1974) (66)	31	48%	39%	Amino acids removed	Haemocol 300, heparin
Silk and Williams (1978) (97)	71	—	23.9%	—	Haemocol 300, heparin
Gelfand et al. (1978) (75)	10	90%	40%	Amino acid B/A ratio rose, csf cAMP rose	Haemocol 300, heparin
Gimson et al. (1982) (69)	31 Grade III	68%	65%	Cerebral oedema 49%	Haemocol 100, heparin
	45 Grade IV	22%	20%	Cerebral oedema 78%	Prostacyclin
Bihari et al. (1983) (78)	13 Grade IV	—	42%	—	XAD-7 albumin-coated resin 360 g
	6 Grade III	—	—	—	
Kennedy et al. (1985) (76)	12 Grade IV	—	33%	Platelets fell 50%	Haemocol 100, heparin

B/A ratio = branched chain/aromatic acid ratio (see text)

TABLE 3.8   Hepatic failure toxins removed with haemoperfusion

Amino acids	Fatty acids – oleic, hexanoic, octanoic
Aromatic > branched chain	N-valeric
(Ammonia)	(Glucose)
Bile acids	Mercaptan
Bilirubin	Middle molecules
(Calcium)	Norepinephrine
Coagulation factors	Octopamine
(Cyclic AMP)	Phenols
Dopamine	Protein-bound molecules
Epinephrine	Inhibitor of Na/K ATPase

() = poorly removed

OTHER USES OF HAEMOPERFUSION

A dramatic improvement in schizophrenic patients treated with haemodialysis has been reported[80]. Treatment techniques such as haemoperfusion and haemofiltration have also been used[81,82] with mixed results. Controlled clinical trials of dialysis in schizophrenia have, however, been inconclusive[83].

Similarly, patients with severe psoriasis treated with peritoneal dialysis and haemodialysis have improved, while others have developed the disease during regular dialysis[84]. Haemoperfusion and haemofiltration[84,85] have also been used to treat severe psoriasis but controlled clinical trials have demonstrated little value[84].

Several authors have attempted to remove chemotherapeutic drugs from patients given high doses, either inadvertently or therapeutically[86]. Initial reports of uncoated charcoal haemoperfusion in removal of methotrexate were encouraging, but subsequent reports of XAD-4 resin or uncoated charcoal haemoperfusion and haemodialysis or peritoneal dialysis have not been promising[87] despite isolated enthusiastic reports[88]. Adriamycin can be removed by charcoal haemoperfusion and drug elimination rates increased substantially[89]. Prolonged haemoperfusion would, however, be required to reduce tissue levels of this drug. Regional haemoperfusion to remove chemotherapeutic drugs after intracarotid infusions for brain tumours, has been used to reduce systemic exposure and consequent side effects in man[90].

Specific adsorption of immune proteins on antigen- or antibody-coated carrier particles in haemoperfusion columns has also been developed. Introduced by Terman and co-workers[91], it is now possible to remove antibodies to such proteins or polypeptides as bovine serum albumin, deoxyribonucleic acid and antiglomerular basement membrane antibody from blood percolated through immuno-adsorbent systems. DNA-collodion coated charcoal haemoperfusion removed single stranded anti-DNA antibodies and immune complexes from the blood of a patient with systemic lupus erythematosus. Subendothelial glomerular deposits were less marked in the renal biopsy obtained after such treatment[92]. In dogs with spontaneous breast cancer, passage of blood over a column containing staphylococcal A protein was associated with regression and complete disappearance of the tumours[93]. Studies of this technique in human cancer are in progress[94]. The technique has also been used to remove poisons by immunoadsorption with successful reversal of digoxin poisoning after haemoperfusion of blood through digoxin antibody-coated poly-acrolein microsphere beads[95]. Haemoperfusion has also been used in the removal of bilirubin[214] and plasma lipids as well as a variety of other conditions, including sepsis, for which its role is not yet defined[96].

FUTURE DEVELOPMENTS IN HAEMOPERFUSION

Treatment of uraemia will probably involve the hybridization of sorbent technology in conjunction with dialysis/haemofiltration. Current interest concerns the removal of middle molecules and urea.

Haemoperfusion is of proven benefit in acute drug intoxication but is less valuable in uraemia and hepatic encephalopathy. Specific extracorporeal immunoadsorbent columns are likely to be developed further. At present, they have a real but relatively minor role in some cases of poisoning (e.g. digoxin). In future they may help to define the role of specific antibodies in mediating certain diseases and perhaps may ultimately prove of value in treating some immune-mediated diseases.

REFERENCES

1. Yatzidis, H. (1964). A convenient haemoperfusion micro-apparatus over charcoal for the treatment of endogenous and exogenous intoxications. Its use as an artifical kidney. *Proc. Eur. Dial. Transplant. Assoc.*, **1**, 83
2. Dunea, G. and Kolff, W. J. (1965). Clinical experience with the Yatzidis charcoal artifical kidney. *Trans. Am. Soc. Artif. Intern. Organs*, **11**, 178
3. Chang, T. M. S. (1966). Semipermeable aqueous microcapsules (artificial cells): with emphasis on experiments in an extracorporeal shunt system. *Trans. Am. Soc. Artif. Intern. Organs*, **12**, 13
4. Denti, E., Luboz, M. P. and Tessore, V. (1975). Adsorption characteristics of cellulose acetate coated charcoals. *J. Biomed. Mater. Res.*, **9**, 143
5. Cornelis, R., Ringoir, S., Mees, L. and Hoste, J. (1980). Behaviour of trace metals during hemoperfusion. *Mineral Electrol. Metab.*, **4**, 123

6. Hagstam, K. E., Larsson, L. E. and Thysell, H. (1966). Experimental studies on charcoal haemoperfusion in phenobarbital intoxication and uraemia, including histopathologic findings. *Acta Med. Scand.*, **180**, 593

7. Winchester, J. F. (1980). Hemoperfusion in uremia. In Giordano, C. (eds.) *Sorbents and Their Clinical Applications*, p. 387. (New York: Academic Press Inc.)

8. Chang, T. M. S. (1978). Microcapsule artificial kidney in replacement of renal function. With emphasis on adsorbent hemoperfusion. In Drukker, W., Parsons, F. M. and Maher, J. F (eds.). *Replacement of Renal Function by Dialysis*, p. 217. First Edition, (The Hague, Boston, London: Martinus Nijhoff Publishers)

9. Stefoni, S., Feliciangeli, G., Coli, L. and Bonomini, V. (1979). Evaluation of a new coated charcoal for hemoperfusion in uremia. *Int. J. Artif. Organs*, **2**, 320

10. Pott, G., Voss, B., Lohmann, J. and Zundorf, P. (1982). Loss of fibronectin in plasma of patients with shock and septicaemia, and after haemoperfusion in patients with severe poisoning. *J. Clin. Chem. Clin. Biochem.*, **20**, 333

11. Winchester, J. F., Ratcliffe, J. G., Carlyle, E. and Kennedy, A. C. (1978). Solute, amino acid, and hormone changes with coated charcoal hemoperfusion in uremia. *Kidney Int.*, **14**, 74

12. Gimson, A. E. S., Langley, P. G., Hughes, R. D, Canalese, J., Mellon, P. G., Williams, R., Woods, H. F. and Weston, M. J. (1980). Prostacyclin to prevent platelet activation during charcoal haemoperfusion in fulminant hepatic failure. *Lancet*, **1**, 173

13. Muirhead, E. E. and Reid, A. F. (1984). Resin artificial kidney. *J. Lab. Clin. Med.*, **33**, 841

14. Yatzidis, H., Voudiclari, S., Oreopoulos, D., Tsaparas, N., Triantaphyllidis, D., Gavras, C. and Stavroulaki, A. (1965). Treatment of severe barbiturate poisoning. *Lancet*, **2**, 216

15. Chang, T. M. S., Gonda, A., Dirks, J. H. and Malave, N. (1971). Clinical evaluation of chronic intermittent and short term hemoperfusion in patients with chronic renal failure using semipermeable microcapsules (artificial cells) formed from membrane coated activated charcoal. *Trans. Am. Soc. Artif. Intern. Organs*, **17**, 246

16. Chang, T. M. S. and Migchelsen, M. (1973) Characterization of possible 'toxic' metabolites in uremia and hepatic coma based on the clearance spectrum for larger molecules by the ACAC microcapsule artificial kidney. *Trans. Am. Soc. Artif. Intern. Organs*, **19**, 314

17. Chang, T. M. S., Migchelsen, M., Coffey, J. F. and Stark, R. (1974). Serum middle molecule levels in uremia during long term intermittent hemoperfusion with ACAC (coated charcoal) microcapsule artificial kidney. *Trans. Am. Soc. Artif. Intern. Organs*, **20**, 364

18. Odaka, M., Hirasawa, H., Kobayashi, H., Ohkawa, M., Soeda, K., Tabata, Y., Soma, M. and Sato, H. (1980). Clinical and fundamental studies of cellulose coated bead-shaped charcoal haemoperfusion in chronic renal failure. In Sideman, S. and Chang, T. M. S. (eds.) Hemoperfusion, Kidney and Liver Support and Detoxification, p. 45. (Washington DC: Hemisphere Publishing Corp.)

19. Trznadel, K., Luciak, M. and Wyszogrodzka, M. (1981). Effect of haemoperfusion on the left ventricular systolic function in patients with chronic uraemia. *Acta Med. Pol.*, **22**, 75

20. Stefoni, S., Coli, L., Feliciangeli, G., Baldrati, L. and Bonomini, V. (1980).

Regular hemoperfusion in regular dialysis treatment. A long-term study. *Int. J. Artif. Organs*, **3**, 348

21. Otsubo, O., Kuzuhara, K., Simada, Y., Yamauchi, Y., Takahashi, I., Yamada, Y., Otsubo, K. and Inou, T. (1979) Treatment of uraemic peripheral neuritis by direct haemoperfusion with activated charcoal. *Proc. Eur. Dial. Transplant Assoc.*, **16**, 731

22. Chang, T. M. S., Barre, P. and Kuruvilla, S. (1985). Long-term reduced time hemoperfusion–hemodialysis compared to standard dialysis. A preliminary cross-over analysis. *Trans. Am. Soc. Artif. Intern. Organs*, **31**, 572

23. Henderson, I. S. and Kennedy, A. C. (1984). Long-term evaluation of charcoal haemoperfusion combined with dialysis for uraemic patients. In Paul, J. P., Gaylor, J. D. S., Courtney, J. M., Gilchrist, T. (eds.) *Biomaterials in Artificial Organs*, p. 72. (London and Basingstoke: The Macmillan Press Ltd.)

24. Bonomini, V., Stefoni, S., Feliciangeli, G., Coli, L., Scolari, M. P., Prandini, R., Casciani, C. U., Taccone Gallucci, Albertazzi, A., Mioli, V., Mastrangelo, F. (1984). Present status of hemoperfusion/hemodialysis in Italy. *Appl. Biochem. Biotechnol.*, **10**, 157

25. Barre, P. E., Gonda, A. and Chang, T. M. S. (1986). Routine clinical applications of hemodialysis-hemoperfusion in chronic renal failure: case reports. *Int. J. Artif. Organs*, **9**, 305

26. Vale, J. A., Meredith, T. and Buckley, B. (1984). ABC of poisoning. Eliminating poisons. *Br. Med. J.*, **289**, 366

27. Litovitz, T. and Veltri, J. (1985). 1984 annual report of the American Association of Poison Control Centers. *Am. J. Emerg. Med.*, **3**, 423

28. Henry, J. A. and Cassidy, S. L. (1986). Membrane stabilising ability: A major cause of fatal poisoning. *Lancet*, **1**, 1414

29. Litovitz, T. L., Normann, S. A. and Veltri, J. C. (1986). 1985 annual report of the American Association of Poison Control Centers National Data Collection System. *Am. J. Emerg. Med.*, **4**, 427

30. Haddad, L. M. (1986). A general approach to poisoning. In Winchester, J. F. (ed.) *Office Procedures: Office Management of Poisoning*, p. 325. (Philadelphia: Hanley and Belfus Inc.)

31. Clemmesen, C. and Nilsson, E. (1961). Therapeutic trends in the treatment of barbiturate poisoning: The Scandinavian method. *Clin. Pharmacol. Ther.*, **2**, 220

32. Winchester, J. F., Gelfand, M. C. and Tilstone, W. J. (1978). Hemoperfusion in drug intoxication – Clinical and laboratory aspects. *Drug Metab. Rev.*, **8**, 69

33. Winchester, J. F., Gelfand, M. C., Knepshield, J. H. and Schreiner, G. E. (1977). Dialysis and hemoperfusion of poisons and drugs – Update. *Trans. Am. Soc. Artif. Intern. Organs*, **23**, 762

34. Rosenbaum, J. L., Kramer, M. S., Raja, R. M., Krug, M. J. and Bolisay, C. G. (1980). Current status of hemoperfusion in toxicology. *Clin. Toxicol*, **17**, 493

35. Winchester, J. F., Tilstone, W. J., Edwards, R. O., Gilchrist, T. and Kennedy, A. C. (1974). Hemoperfusion for enhanced drug elimination – A kinetic analysis in paracetamol poisoning. *Trans. Am. Soc. Artif. Intern. Organs*, **20**, 358

36. Pond, S., Rosenberg, J., Benowitz, N. L. and Takki, S. (1979). Pharmacokinetics of haemoperfusion in drug overdose. *Clin. Pharmacokinet.*, **4**, **329**

37. Cutler, R. E., Forland, S. C., St John Hammond, P. G. and Evans, R. J. (1987). Extracorporeal removal of drugs and poisons by hemodialysis and hemoperfusion. *Ann. Rev. Pharmacol. Toxicol.*, **27**, 169

38. Lorch, J. A. and Garella, S. (1979). Hemoperfusion to treat intoxications. *Ann. Intern. Med.*, **91**, 301
39. Uldall, P. R. (1982). Controlled trial of resin hemoperfusion for the treatment of drug overdose at Toronto Western Hospital (TWH). *Trans. Am. Soc. Artif. Intern. Organs*, **28**, 676
40. Winchester, J. F. (1983). Active methods for detoxification: Oral sorbents, forced diuresis, hemoperfusion, and hemodialysis. In Haddad, L. M. and Winchester, J. F. (eds.) *Clinical Management of Poisoning and Drug Overdose*, p. 154. (Philadelphia: W. B. Saunders Co.)
41. Gazzard, B. G., Willson, R. A., Weston, M. J., Thompson, R. and Williams, R., (1974). Charcoal haemoperfusion for paracetamol overdose. *Br. J. Clin. Pharmacol.*, **1**, 217
42. Winchester, J. F., Gelfand, M. C., Helliwell, M., Vale, J. A., Goulding, R. and Schreiner, G. E. (1981). Extracorporeal treatment of salicylate or acetaminophen poisoning – Is there a role? *Arch. Intern. Med.*, **141**, 370
43. Diaz-Buxo, J. A., Farmer, C. D. and Chandler, T. Y. (1978). Hemoperfusion in the treatment of amitriptyline poisoning. *Trans. Am. Soc. Artif. Intern. Organs*, **24**, 699
44. Trafford, J. A. P., Jones, R. H., Evans, R., Sharp, P., Sharpstone, P. and Cook, J. (1977). Haemoperfusion with R-004 amberlite resin for treating acute poisoning. *Br. Med. J.*, **2**, 1453
45. Crome, P., Braithwaite, R. A., Widdop, B. and Medd, R. K. (1980). Haemoperfusion in clinical and experimental tricyclic antidepressant poisoning. In Sideman, S. and Chang, T. M. S. (eds.) *Hemoperfusion, Kidney and Liver Support and Detoxification*, p. 301. (Washington DC: Hemisphere Publishing Corp.)
46. Hoy, W. E., Gibson, T. P., Rivero, A. J., Jain, J. K., Talley, T. T., Bayer, R. M., Montondo, D. F. and Freeman, R. B. (1983). XAD-4 resin hemoperfusion for digitoxic patients with renal failure. *Kidney Int.*, **23**, 79
47. Wenger, T. L., Butler, V. P. Jr, Haber, E. and Smith, T. W. (1985). Treatment of 63 severely digitalis-toxic patients with digoxin specific antibody fragments. *J. Am. Coll. Cardiol.*, **5**, (5 Suppl A), 118A
48. Maini, R. and Winchester, J. F. (1975). Removal of paraquat from blood by haemoperfusion over sorbent materials. *Br. Med. J.*, **3**, 281
49. Mascie-Taylor, B. H., Thompson, J. and Davison, A. M. (1983). Haemoperfusion ineffective for paraquat removal in life-threatening poisoning. *Lancet*, **1**, 1376
50. Okonek, S., Baldamus, C. A., Hofman, A., Schuster, C. J., Bechstein, P. B. and Zoller, B. (1979). Two survivors of severe paraquat intoxication by 'continuous hemoperfusion.' *Klin. Wochenshr.*, **57**, 957
51. Gelfand, M. C., Winchester, J. F., Knepshield, J. H., Hanson, K. M., Cohan, S. L., Strauch, B. S., Geoly, K. L., Kennedy, A. C. and Schreiner, G. E. (1977). Treatment of severe drug overdose with charcoal hemoperfusion. *Trans. Am. Soc. Artif. Intern. Organs*, **23**, 599
52. Connell, J. M., McGeachie, J. F., Knepil, J., Thomson, A. and Junor, B. (1982). Self-poisoning with sustained-release aminophylline: secondary rise in serum theophylline concentration after charcoal haemoperfusion. *Br. Med. J.*, **284**, 943
53. Ahlmen, J., Heath, A., Herlitz, H., Kvist, L. and Mellstrand, T. (1984). Treatment of oral theophylline poisoning. *Acta Med. Scand.*, **216**, 423
54. Chang, T. M. S. and Barre, P. (1983). Effect of desferrioxamine on removal of

aluminium and iron by coated charcoal haemoperfusion and haemodialysis. *Lancet*, **2**, 1051

55. Winchester, J. F. (1986). Management of iron overload. *Semin. Nephrol.*, **4**, (suppl. 1), 22

56. Andress, D. L., Maloney, N. A., Endres, D. B. and Sherrard, D. J. (1986). Aluminium-associated bone disease in chronic renal failure: high prevalence in a long-term dialysis population. *J. Bone Miner. Res.*, **1**, 391

57. Arieff, A. I. (1985). Aluminium and the pathogenesis of dialysis encephalopathy. *Am. J. Kidney Dis.*, **6**, 317

58. Bregman, H., Gelfand, M. C., Winchester, J. F., Manz, H. J., Knepshield, J. H. and Schreiner, G. E. (1980). Iron overload-associated myopathy in patients on maintenance haemodialysis. A histocompatibility linked disorder. *Lancet*, **2**, 882

59. Marcus, R. E., Davies, S. C., Bantock, H. M., Underwood, S. R., Walton, S. and Huehns, E. R. (1984). Desferrioxamine to improve cardiac function in iron overloaded patients with thalassemia major. *Lancet*, **1**, 392

60. Lund, M. E., Banner, W., Clarkson, T. W. and Berlin, M. (1984). Treatment of acute methylmercury ingestion by hemodialysis with *n*-acetylcysteine (Mucomyst) infusion and 2,3-dimercaptopropane sulfonate. *J. Toxicol. Clin. Toxicol*, **22**, 31

61. Al-Abassi, A. H., Kostyniak, P. J. and Clarkson, T. W. (1978). An extracorporeal complexing hemodialysis system for the treatment of methylmercury poisoning. III Clinical applications. *J. Pharmacol. Exp. Ther.*, **207**, 249

62. Margel, S. (1981). A novel approach for heavy metal poisoning treatment, a model. Mercury poisoning by means of chelating microspheres; hemoperfusion and oral administration. *J. Med. Chem.*, **24**, 1263

63. James, J. H., Ziparo, V., Jeppson, B. and Fischer, J. E. (1979). Hyperammonaemia, plasma aminoacid imbalance, and blood–brain aminoacid transport: A unified theory of portal-systemic encephalopathy. *Lancet*, **2**, 772

64. Schafer, D. F. and Jones, E. A. (1982). Hepatic encephalopathy and the gamma-aminobutyric-acid neurotransmitter system. *Lancet*, **1**, 18

65. Chang, T. M. S. (1972). Haemoperfusion over microencapsulated adsorbent in a patient with hepatic coma. *Lancet*, **2**, 1371

66. Gazzard, B. G., Portmann, B. A., Weston, M. J., Langley, P. G., Murray-Lyon, I. M., Dunlop, E. H., Flax, H., Mellon, P. J., Record, C. O., Ward, M. B. and Williams, R. (1974). Charcoal haemoperfusion in the treatment of fulminant hepatic failure. *Lancet*, **1**, 1301

67. Silk, D. B. A. and Williams, R. (1980). Sorbents in hepatic failure. In Giordano, C. (ed.) *Sorbents and Their Clinical Applications*, p. 415. (New York: Academic Press Inc.)

68. Chang, T. M. S., Lister, C., Chirito, E., O'Keefe, P., Resurreccion, E. (1978). Effects of hemoperfusion rate and time of initiation of ACAC charcoal hemoperfusion on the survival of fulminant hepatic failure rats. *Trans. Am. Soc. Artif. Intern. Organs*, **24**, 243

69. Gimson, A. E. S., Braude, S., Mellon, P. J., Canalese, J. and Williams, R. (1982). Earlier charcoal haemoperfusion in fulminant hepatic failure. *Lancet*, **2**, 681

70. Tygstrup, N. and Ranek, L. (1986). Fulminant hepatic failure. *Clin. Gastroenterol.*, **10**, 191

71. Hughes, R. D., Cochrane, A. M. D., Thomson, A. D., Murray-Lyon and

79

Williams, R. (1976). Cytotoxicity of plasma from patients with acute hepatic failure to isolated rabbit hepatocytes. *Br. J. Exp. Pathol.*, **57**, 348

72. Seda, H. W. M., Hughes, R. D., Give, C. D. and Williams, R. (1984). Removal of inhibitors of brain Na⁺ K⁺ ATPase by haemoperfusion in fulminant hepatic failure. *Artif. Organs*, **8**, 174

73. Woods, H. F., Weston, M. J., Bunting, S., Moncada, S. and Vane, J. (1980). Prostacyclin eliminates the thrombocytopenia associated with charcoal hemoperfusion and minimizes heparin and fibrinogen consumption. *Artif. Organs*, **4**, 176

74. Rubin, M. H., Weston, M. J., Bullock, G., Roberts, J., Langley, P. G., White, Y. S. and Williams, R. (1977). Abnormal platelet function and ultrastructure in fulminant hepatic failure. *Q. J. Med.*, **46**, 339

75. Gelfand, M. C., Winchester, J. F., Knepshield, J. H., Cohan, S.I. and Schreiner, G. E. (1978). Reversal of hepatic coma by coated charcoal hemoperfusion: Clinical and biochemical observations. asaio J., **1**, 73

76. Kennedy, H. J., Greaves, M. and Triger, D. R. (1985). Clinical experience with the use of charcoal haemoperfusion: Is prostacyclin required? *Life Support Syst.*, **3**, 115

77. Berk, P. D. (1977). A computer simulation study relating to the treatment of fulminant hepatic failure by hemoperfusion. *Proc. Soc. Exp. Biol. Med.*, **155**, 535

78. Bihari, D., Hughes, R. D., Gimson, A. E. S., Langley, P. G., Ede, R. J., Eder, G. and Williams, R. (1983). Effects of serial resin haemoperfusion in fulminant hepatic failure. *Int. J. Artif. Organs*, **6**, 299

79. Hughes, R. and Williams, R. (1986). Clinical experience with charcoal and resin hemoperfusion. *Semin. Liver Dis.*, **6**, 164

80. Wagemaker, H. and Cade, R. (1977). The use of hemodialysis in chronic schizophrenia. *Am. J. Psychiatr.*, **134**, 684

81. Chang, T. M. S. (1978). Hemoperfusion in chronic schizophrenia. *Int. J. Artif. Organs*, **1**, 253.

82. Nedipil, N., Dieterle, D. and Gurland, H. Y. (1980). Blood purification treatment of schizophrenia. *Int. J. Artif. Organs*, **3**, 76

83. Schulz, S. C., VanKammen, D. P., Balow, J. E., Flye, N. W. and Bunney, W. E. (1981). Dialysis in schizophrenia: A double blind evaluation. *Science*, **211**, 1066

84. Nissensson, A. B., Rapaport, M., Gordon, A. and Narins, R. G. (1978). Controlled study demonstrates that psoriasis is not improved by haemodialysis. *Kidney Int.*, **14**, 682

85. Maeda, K., Asada, H., Yamamoto, Y. and Ohta, K. (1980). Psoriasis treatment with direct hemoperfusion. In Sideman, S. and Chang, T. M. S. (eds.) *Hemoperfusion, Kidney and Liver Support and Detoxification*, p. 349. (Washington DC: Hemisphere Publishing Corp.)

86. Winchester, J. F., Rahman, A., Bregman, H., Mortensen, L. M., Gelfand, M. C., Schein, P. S. and Schreiner, G. E. (1980). Role of hemoperfusion in anticancer drug removal. In Sideman, S. and Chang, T. M. S. (eds.) *Hemoperfusion, Kidney and Liver Support and Detoxification*, p. 369. (Washingon DC: Hemisphere Publishing Corp.)

87. Hande, K. R., Balow, J. E., Draje, J. C., Rosenberg, S. A. and Chabner, B. A. (1977). Methotrexate and hemodialysis. *Ann. Intern. Med.*, **87**, 496

88. Molina, R., Fabian, C. and Cowley, B. Jr (1987). Use of charcoal hemoperfusion

to reduce serum methotrexate levels in a patient with acute renal insufficiency. *Am. J. Med.*, **82,** 350

89. Winchester, J. F., Rahman, A., Tilstone, W. J., Kessler, A., Mortensen, L., Schreiner, G. E. and Schein, P. S. (1979). Sorbent removal of adriamycin in vitro and in vivo. *Cancer Treat. Rep.*, **63,** 1787

90. Oldfield, E. H., Dedrick, R. L., Yeager, R. L., Clark, W. C., DeVroom, H. L., Chatterji, D. C. and Doppman, J. L. (1985). Reduced systemic drug exposure by continuous intra-arterial chemotherapy with hemoperfusion of regional venous drainage. *J. Neurosurg.*, **163,** 726–732

91. Terman, D. S. (1980). Extracorporeal immunoadsorbents for extraction of circulation immune reactants. In Giordano, C. (ed.) *Sorbents and Their Clinical Applications*, p. 470. (New York: Academic Press Inc.)

92. Terman, D. S., Buffaloe, G., Mattioli, C., Cook, G., Tillquist, R., Sullivan, M. and Ayus, J. C. (1979). Extracorporeal immunoabsorption: Initial experience in human systemic lupus erythematosus. *Lancet*, **2,** 824

93. Terman, D. S., Yamamoto, T., Mattioli, M., Cook, G., Tillquis, R., Henry, J., Poser and Daskal, Y. (1980). Extensive necrosis of spontaneous canine mammary adenocarcinoma after extracorporeal perfusion over staphylococcus aureus Cowans I. *J. Immunol.*, **124,** 795

94. Terman, D. S. and Bertram, J. H. (1985). Antitumor effects of immobilized protein A and Staphylococcal products: Linkage between toxicity and efficacy and tumoricidal reagents. *Eur. J. Cancer Clin. Oncol.*, **21,** 1115

95. Savin, H., Marcus, L., Margel, S., Ofarim, M. and Ravid, M. (1987). Treatment of adverse digitalis effects of hemoperfusion through columns with antidigoxin antibodies bound to agarose polyacrolein microsphere beads. *Am. Heart J.*, **113,** 1078

96. Chang, T. M. S. and Nicolaev, V. G. (1987). Hemoperfusion, sorbents and immobilized bioreactants. *Biomater. Artif. Cells Artif. Organs*, **15,** (special issue)

97. Silk, D. B. A. and Williams, R. (1978). Experiences in the treatment of fulminant hepatic failure by conservative therapy, charcoal haemoperfusion and polyacrylonitrile haemodialysis. *Int. J. Artif. Organs*, **1,** 29

4
ANTICOAGULATION FOR HAEMODIALYSIS

I. S. HENDERSON

INTRODUCTION

Since the earliest description of vividiffusion (or haemodialysis), clotting of blood on the colloidin membrane has been recorded as a problem[1]. The anticoagulant used to prevent this phenomenon in the earliest experiments was leech head extract and a method was described for producing a usable solution of this substance called hirudin[2]. Availability and toxicity of these preparations remained a problem until 1937[3] when the use of heparin as an anticoagulant for haemodialysis was described[4].

Heparin today remains the mainstay of anticoagulation for haemodialysis and this chapter will review the principles and practices relating to its use and the development of alternative drugs and methods of anticoagulation.

Initially, it will be necessary to review the haemostatic system, tests of its function and the events which follow the interaction of blood with foreign surfaces.

THE HAEMOSTATIC SYSTEM

General description

Damage to vascular endothelium or contact of blood with a 'foreign' surface induces a very rapid local haemostatic reaction. Exposure of subendothelial substances (especially collagen) with which blood is not normally in contact induces platelet adherence and secretion of the contents of granules contained in platelet cytoplasm (notably ADP, serotonin and platelet factor IV). Platelet membrane phospholipids are released and metabolized into thromboxane A_2 which promotes further platelet aggregation and activation. A platelet plug is thus formed. While the platelet plug is formed, the blood clotting cascade is activated via a tissue factor which initiates the extrinsic system and surface activation of factor XII which initiates the intrinsic system. The final common pathway of both systems is to activate prothrombin to thrombin which catalyses the breakdown of fibrinogen to fibrin monomer which polymerizes and then crosslinks, resulting in an insoluble clot. The platelet–fibrin mass (often containing red cells) contracts and forms a thrombus – this is due in part to the contractile properties of platelets.

The coagulation system is controlled by a series of inhibitors of the coagulation factors, the most important of which are antithrombin III, C1 inhibitor (shared with the complement system) and protein C. The locally initiated clotting cascade does not become generalized because of these circulating inhibitors which are less effective locally – many of the coagulation factors are adsorbed on to platelet membranes and are resistant to attack there. The other major defence against uncontrolled coagulation is the fibrinolytic system where plasmin, a proteolytic enzyme (activated by intrinsic or contact activation and extrinsic or tissue damage systems), lyses fibrin. This process, in turn, is regulated by circulating antiplasmins. Both coagulation and fibrinolysis must be in dynamic equilibrium to maintain blood vessel patency.

84

Intrinsic and extrinsic cascades (Figure 4.1)

In the intrinsic system, exposed subendothelial tissues, espcially collagen, bind and activate factor XII. Kallikrein and high molecular weight kininogen are involved in the activation process. Factor XIIa

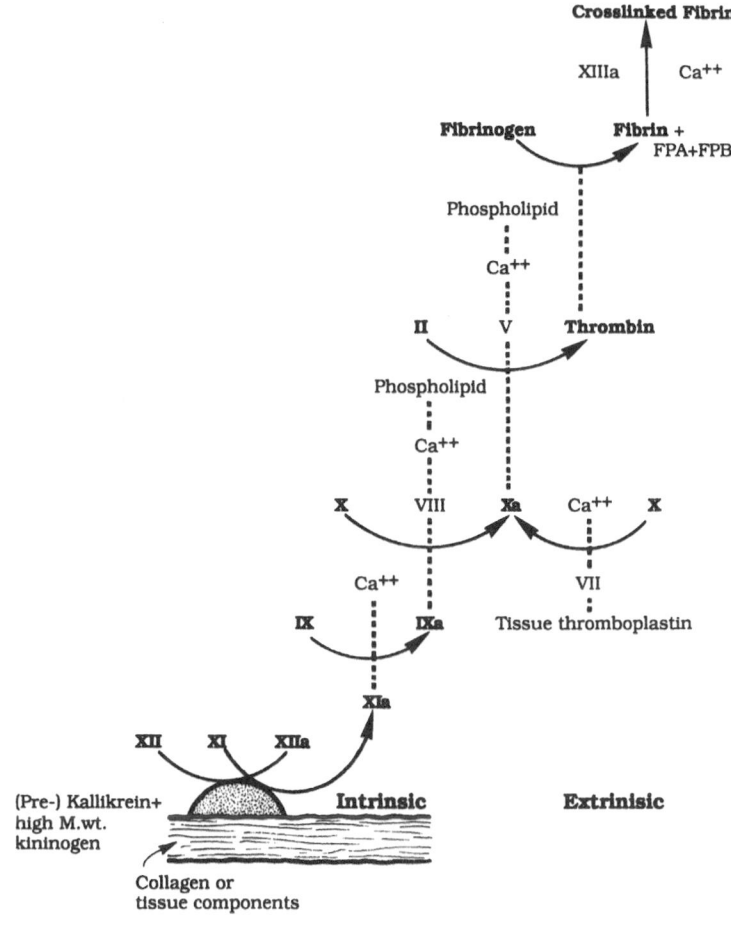

FIGURE 4.1   Intrinsic and extrinsic clotting cascades

activates factor XI which activates factor IX (calcium dependent). In the presence of platelet membrane phospholipids, factor VIII and calcium, factor IXa catalyses the activation of factor X. Factor Xa binds to factor V and platelet phospholipids in the presence of calcium – a complex which facilitates conversion of prothrombin to thrombin (IIa). Thrombin has a strong augmenting effect on the actions of factors V and VIII.

In the extrinsic system, tissue thromboplastin, derived from damaged subendothelial tissue, activated white cells and damaged endothelial cells, complexes with factor VII leading to the activation of factor X in the presence of calcium.

Thereafter, both intrinsic and extrinsic systems share a common pathway. Thrombin splits fibrinogen into monomeric fibrin and fibrinopeptides A and B. Fibrin monomers polymerize and factor XIII (activated by thrombin) catalyses crosslinkage in the presence of calcium to form an insoluble clot. Other actions of thrombin include promotion of platelet aggregation and secretion.

Circulating inhibitors modify the activity of the clotting factors. The most important of these is antithrombin III, an alpha II globulin, which complexes irreversibly with factors XIIa, XIa, Xa and IIa. Its action is markedly increased by heparin. Protein C inhibits factors V and VIII.

Platelets activated by ADP or collagen accelerate activation of factors XII and XI in the presence of kallikrein. Factor XII thus activated probably remains associated with the platelet and is resistant to inactivation. Platelet membrane phospholipids are also important in accelerating activation of factors X and II. Factor VIII Von Willebrand activity (VIIIvWa) is important in mediating the interaction of platelets with surfaces. All plasma procoagulants, except VIII (which originates in the endothelium), are synthesized in the liver. Factors II, VII, IX and X are vitamin K dependent.

The fibrinolytic system

There is a series of circulating and tissue activators and inhibitors of fibrinolysis. In the intrinsic system, XIIa catalyses the activation of plasminogen proactivator. In the extrinsic system, an as yet poorly-defined tissue activator of plasminogen is produced. Streptokinase and urokinase act in a similar manner.

Plasmin can be generated both on the surface of fibrin and free in plasma. In the former case, all the components of the reaction are firmly bound to fibrin, important in limiting the systemic effects of plasmin, a potent proteolytic enzyme which will attack fibrinogen, factors VIII, V and complement. Alpha II antiplasmin neutralizes circulating plasmin but fibrin-bound plasmin is protected.

Platelet function and interaction with surfaces

Platelets are anucleate discoid-shaped cells derived from mega-karyocytes. A substantial proportion of platelets is sequestered in the spleen and the average lifespan is a little over a week. Synthesis of platelets may increase tenfold during demand. Platelets react con-sistently when activated – a process labelled the basic platelet reaction.

Platelets may be activated by ADP, adrenaline, serotonin, surface-bound or aggregated IgG, arachidonate, prostaglandin endoperoxides PGG_2 and PGH_2, thromboxane A_2, collagen and thrombin, each with a specific receptor. These activators have been classified into weak, strong or intermediate on the basis of the degree of reaction triggered. All act through the same intracellular final messenger, probably ionized calcium. Weak activators induce only enough calcium release to cause aggregation and shape change; intermediate activators (e.g. thromboxane A_2) do this but also induce release of dense granule contents and arachidonate. A strong inducer (e.g. thrombin) in addition will liberate the contents of alpha granules.

The basic platelet reaction starts with induction by the activator via a specific receptor leading to transmission – the appearance of the intracellular messenger – ionized calcium. The executive phase com-mences with shape change from discoid to spherical and generation of adhesiveness followed by aggregation (fibrinogen is reversibly bound to the platelet membrane and crosslinks, again reversibly, via calcium bridges, leading to aggregation). The third stage of the executive phase is release of ADP, ATP and serotonin from dense granules. The final stage involves release of alpha granule contents including β-thromboglobulin and platelet factor IV. During the third

87

stage, membrane arachidonate is hydrolysed from phospholipids catalysed by thrombin-specific phospholipase C on inositolphospholipids and phospholipase A_2 on phosphatidylcholine. Free arachidonate is oxidized by cyclo-oxygenase to prostaglandin endoperoxides which are transformed into thromboxane A_2 (Figure 4.2). All these substances are potent platelet activators. Aspirin and non-steroidal antiinflammatory agents block oxidation of arachidonate and cyclic AMP inhibits production of arachidonate and epoprostenol stimulates adenylate cyclase increasing levels of cyclic AMP. Epoprostenol which is produced from cyclic endoperoxides PGG_2 and PGH_2 by an endothelial-derived enzyme (prostacyclin synthetase) is one of the major factors opposing platelet activation. When platelets are activated by contact with artificial surfaces, there is unopposed production of TxA_2. The interaction of platelets with artifical surfaces is probably mediated

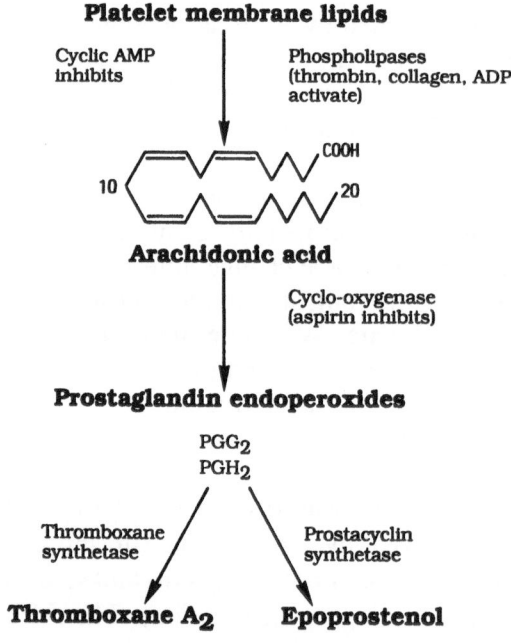

FIGURE 4.2 Synthetic pathways of thromboxane and epoprostenol

via a coating of plasma proteins. Protein adsorption on to the surface precedes platelet adhesion and further activation.

The proportions in which clots on surfaces are composed of platelets or fibrin depends on the surface and the pattern of blood flow. High or turbulent blood flow favours predominantly white or platelet thrombi.

Assessment of blood coagulation for dialysis purposes

In this section, only a brief review will be undertaken of tests of value to monitor coagulation in uraemia and routine anticoagulation with heparin in haemodialysis. More details can be found in textbooks and the review by Lindsay[9].

Whole blood clotting time (WBCT)

Clean glass test tubes are filled with 1 ml of blood taken by vene-puncture through a standard 21 guage needle, covered and rotated gently at 37°C until clotting occurs, usually in around 5 minutes. After dialysis is commenced, the WBCT is monitored at regular intervals; sufficient heparin is administered to the patient to prolong the test to 10–20 min. This test cannot achieve sufficient flexibility to allow rapid alterations in heparin dosage but it will continue to be used as the simplest, cheapest and (performed properly) most reproducible clinical control for heparin requirement.

Whole blood activated clotting time (WBACT)

The WBACT is a more rapid method of assessing WBCT. The clotting process is accelerated using a high-surface-area surface activator, such as kaolin or ground glass. This normally accelerates the WBCT around three fold, normal values being 100 s, or 250 s during dialysis. The method is simple, reproducible[5] and easily automated[6]. Commercially available devices exist for bedside use and facilitate control of heparin administration.

Partial thromboplastin time (PTT)

Whole blood activated partial thromboplastin time (WBAPTT)

PTT assesses the intrinsic system of coagulation. Plasma is activated with kaolin and cephalin is used as a platelet phospholipid substitute. The test can also be applied to whole blood and automated (WBAPTT). As with the WBACT, simple bedside equipment has been produced to perform the test which has proved a useful and reproducible monitor of heparinization status[5,7,8].

Prothrombin time (PT)

Prothrombin time is the time to clotting after administration of tissue activator to plasma. It evaluates factors I, II, V, VII and X, the extrinsic system. It will be prolonged by heparin.

Thrombin time (TT)

Thrombin time detects solely the conversion of fibrinogen to fibrin and will detect inhibitors of this process, including heparin. Reptilase, used instead of thrombin, is unaffected by heparin and forms the basis of a useful coagulation test. Recent thrombin activity can be detected by assay of the fibrinogen cleavage product, fibrinopeptide A.

Fibrinogen and degradation products (FDP)

Fibrinogen can be assayed chemically. Its degradation products (and those of fibrin) can also be measured and provide an index of plasmin activity.

Assessment of platelet function

Again, in this section, only very basic information relevant to later parts of the chapter will be presented. More detailed information can be found in major coagulation texts.

Whole blood platelet count

Automated methods are now available for counting platelets which should number more than 150 000/ml.

Bleeding time

A small standardized skin incision is made and the time to cessation of bleeding is noted. This is the major *in vivo* test of platelet function and numbers. It only becomes significantly prolonged when platelet counts fall below 50 000/ml. A practical decision on whether to administer platelets would be more influenced by spontaneous bleeding episodes.

Platelet aggregation and platelet specific proteins

Platelet aggregation can be measured in a suspension or in whole blood[10]. Aggregation is usually induced by ADP, collagen or thrombin and quantitated by nephelometry in platelet-rich and platelet-depleted samples. Results can be expressed as aggregation rate or platelet numbers as a fraction of control in a given time. Platelet-specific proteins, including β-thromboglobulin and platelet factor IV can be measured immunologically and provide an index of activity.

ANTICOAGULATION FOR HAEMODIALYSIS

General considerations

One of the major problems in defining an ideal anticoagulant for haemodialysis is that uraemic patients have a bleeding tendency[11-13]. In acute renal failure, disseminated intravascular coagulation is frequently present and relates to the underlying cause of renal failure. In chronic uraemia, the defects are more subtle. Some patients are deficient in factors V and VII[14]; most patients exhibit disordered platelet function leading to diminished aggregation and adhesiveness and a prolonged bleeding time[15]. Some may be thrombocytopaenic.

Institution of regular haemodialysis has been found to improve platelet function[15-19], suggesting dialytic removal of toxins suppressing platelet formation and inhibiting function. Some defects, however, still remain, suggesting larger non-dialysable toxins (in this context Gallice et al.[20] have reviewed the inhibitory effects of 'middle molecules' on platelet aggregation) or other defects not modified by dialysis, including decreased factor VIII – Von Willebrand activity[21], although more recent studies contradict this[22].

There is a considerable body of evidence to suggest that uraemic patients established on haemodialysis may become hypercoagulable, as evidenced by the frequent occurrence of thrombotic[23-25] and thromboembolic events[26]. The possible causes are not fully understood – platelet activity may be enhanced in vivo[23-29] and in vitro platelet aggregation tests may be normal[30,31], increased[32-34] or decreased[18,35,36]. Vaziri et al.[22] has documented increased activities of clotting factors VII, VIII and X and decreased activity of antithrombin III. Platelet activation by the dialyser membrane or the arteriovenous fistula[23,24], as well as heparin therapy[37], have been implicated in platelet hyperactivity in haemodialysis.

Requirement for dialysis anticoagulation

When a dialysis membrane comes into contact with blood, there is protein deposition[38], platelet activation and stimulation of the coagulation cascades. The complement pathway is activated[39], particularly by new (i.e. first-use) cuprophane dialysers whose cellulose residues activate C_{3a} and C_{5a} of the alternative pathway. Reused dialysers have a fine coating of fibrin and other plasma proteins and are less active[40]. Leukocytes also adhere to dialysis membranes[41] and may further stimulate coagulation. Both complement components and leukocyte products may further stimulate platelet aggregability[42]. Although some dialysis membranes are more 'biocompatible' than others[39], anticoagulation of some kind is required to prevent deposition of platelets and fibrin on the dialysis membrane. There has been one report[43] on the use of a hollow fibre cuprophane dialyser in 6 patients without administration of heparin (other than during priming) and using intermittent saline flushes of the dialyser half-hourly during dialysis. Casati *et al.* have also shown that heparin-free dialysis is possible although sometimes very low doses of heparin are required because of partial clotting of the dialyser[44].

SPECIFIC DIALYSIS ANTICOAGULANT DRUGS

In this section, most consideration will be given to the use of heparin, still regarded as the universal anticoagulant for haemodialysis.

Heparin

Structure and actions

Heparin was discovered in 1916 by McLean, three years after the initial vividiffusion experiments. The original preparations were toxic and it was not until 20 years later that a formulation suitable for human administration became available[45].

Heparin is an acidic anionic sulphated mucopolysaccharide of variable molecular weight. It is a polymer of alternating residues of mainly iduronic acid and *N*-acetyl-glucosamine. Its structure is made up of regular sequences of blocks of trisulphated disaccharides interrupted by other hexose moieties which are often less densely sulphated. Approximately one third of the heparin chains contain a specific pentasaccharide sequence which is responsible for high-affinity binding to certain positively charged lysyl residues on antithrombin III. Commercially available heparin solutions contain a normal distribution of heparin molecules of varying size, sulphation and charge.

The main effect exerted by heparin on coagulation is by combination with antithrombin III which is then potentiated in its irreversible inactivation of factors XII, XI, IX, X and II. Another co-factor – heparin cofactor II (HC-II) – which complexes with thrombin has been described but much higher heparin dosage is needed, casting some doubt on the clinical significance[46]. Heparin also binds directly to thrombin. Heparin will inactivate factors IXa, Xa and XIa at one tenth of the dose required to inhibit the other pro-coagulants, which is useful for minimal intermittent heparinization[47,48].

Heparin has a complex interaction with platelets. *In vitro*, it will enhance aggregation induced by ADP: higher molecular weight fractions are more active in this context[49]. *In vivo*, heparin reduces binding of factors IXa and VIII to platelet phospholipids and the binding of thrombin and factor Xa to platelet membranes is inhibited[45]. This renders more Xa available for inactivation by the heparin-AT III complex.

Use in haemodialysis

Inducing adequate anticoagulation for haemodialysis represents a difficult tightrope between, on the one hand, clotting of blood in the extracorporeal circuit with resultant inefficiency of dialysis and blood loss and, on the other, induction of haemorrhagic problems, especially in patients with acute renal failure. It is also important to note that determination of the ideal heparin dosage schedule at the outset of regular dialysis therapy is not enough – it should be redetermined at regular intervals as platelet function may vary with degree of control of uraemia and different dialysis membranes may have very different biocompatibilities. Single needle dialysis also requires more heparin[50].

At least two different regimens exist for heparin administration – intermittent and continuous[51]. Of the two, continuous administration is more likely to maintain a constant blood level of heparin but is less practicable and more expensive as infusion equipment is required. Single-dose heparin for haemodialysis has been used but carries the disadvantages of being difficult to control, leading either to over-anticoagulation and the risk of bleeding or unacceptably low herapin levels towards the end of dialysis leading to clotting complications or unacceptable fibrin deposition on dialysis membranes[52].

Control of heparinization for either continuous or intermittent administration is crucial. There are several methods available. As whole blood clotting time (usually Lee White method – LWBCT) is time consuming and inflexible, one of the activated methods should be used. Whole blood activated clotting time (WBACT) and whole blood activated partial thromboplastin time (WBAPTT) are reproducible, automated and rapid. Rapid assays to measure heparin chemically (using Azure A or B) have now been described and may ultimately replace, or be used in conjunction with, the other tests which monitor heparin activity[53,54].

Detailed pharmacokinetic mathematical models have been developed by Gotch and Keen[55], Farrell et al.[56] and Khazine and Simons[57] to accurately predict heparin requirements calculated from response and sensitivity to heparin.

For practical purposes, Mingardi et al.[51] recommends hourly dosage with heparin aiming to maintain a clotting time of 1.5 to 2 times predialysis values. In practice, this meant 45 iu heparin/kg loading dose, 60% of this value at 1 and 2 hours and 30% at each subsequent hour. For continuous heparin infusion, our own practice is to give a loading dose of 2500 iu heparin and 1250 iu/hour, coupled with hourly assessment of clotting time. If the clotting time exceeds 40 min (180 s WBACT), the infusion rate is reduced by 250 iu/hour and clotting checked half-hourly and adjusted to maintain clotting time in the region of 25–40 min. Should clotting times be greater than 40 min for the entire dialysis, the loading and constant infusion doses are halved for the next dialysis. The converse is true for low clotting times.

For patients at high risk of bleeding, some form of minimal heparinization is required. Williman et al.[47] recommends dosage based on measurement of activated partial thromboplastin time (APTT). Swartz[58] has shown that bleeding in a high-risk uraemic group did not correlate well with amount of heparin used and recommends that enough heparin should be used to prevent dialyser fibrin deposition. The best practical advice is to use as 'biocompatible' a dialyser as possible and to perform frequent (half-hourly) clotting times aiming to maintain 10–15 min[9].

Regional heparinization[59,60] where only the dialyser circuit is anticoagulated, the heparin being neutralized with protamine sulphate before the extracorporeal blood is returned to the patient, has been advocated as theoretically better than continuous heparinization of the patient. However, there is no evidence that bleeding complications are reduced[61]. There may even be a post-dialysis 'rebound' systemic anticoagulation, partly due to dissociation of the heparin protamine complex, the longer halflife of heparin and the intrinsic anticoagulant activity of high doses of protamine. Largely of historical interest for haemodialysis, regional heparinization has recently been successfully used in continuous arteriovenous haemofiltration (CAVH) where patients may be exposed to heparin for long periods of time[62].

Adverse effects

The occurrence of thrombocytopenia is increasingly reported[44] with prolonged use of heparin in patients with normal renal function but is relatively rare in haemodialysis patients[63-65]. Its aetiology is not certain, possibly being related to a heparin-dependent platelet aggregating fator in the IgG fraction of serum. It is noted more often with heparin preparations of bovine rather than porcine origin[66-68]. The platelet aggregation in this condition is associated with activation of the platelet prostaglandin pathway and can be inhibited by inhibitors of prostaglandin synthetase[69,70]. The condition will often resolve on cessation of heparin.

Increased platelet aggregation and depressed levels of antithrombin III post-dialysis (independent phenomena)[22,23] lead to a hypercoagulable state which may explain the increased incidence of thrombotic[22-25] and thromboembolic[26] events in dialysis patients. Heparin has been implicated in the aetiology.

Patients with established haemorrhage are liable to experience further bleeding complications with heparin[58] and, in addition, other bleeding complications have been described, including subdural haematoma[73], haemorrhagic pericarditis[74], intraperitoneal bleeding[74] and haemorrhagic pleural effusions[76].

Other side effects of heparin, including allergy, alopecia and osteoporosis[77], are rare and will not be considered further here. Heparin also induces changes in lipid metabolism by stimulating lipoprotein lipase[78].

Alternative anticoagulants for haemodialysis

Although widely used, heparin cannot be regarded as the ideal anti-coagulant for haemodialysis, because of difficulty in monitoring its effects and the increased tendency to thrombosis and thrombo-embolism post-treatment – due, at least in part, to increased platelet aggregation. Side effects, including bleeding in at-risk patients, have also stimulated the search for a more suitable alternative anticoagulant therapy.

Low molecular weight heparinoids

Smaller molecular weight fragments of heparin also exhibit anti-coagulant properties. The minimum chain length still able to bind to anti-thrombin III is a pentasaccharide[45]. This will inhibit activated factor X but, unlike heparin, appears to be unable to accelerate the inhibitory effect of antithrombin III on thrombin. The effects on factors XI and IX are reduced. It has also been shown that the low molecular weight fractions have less platelet-aggregatory effects[49,79,80]. These properties should lead to preservation of antithrombotic effects with effective reduction in bleeding complications. There are several commercial preparations which are produced by either heparinase or nitrous acid depolymerization of heparin.

The first use of low molecular weight heparinoids in (acute) haemo-dialysis was described by Henny et al.[81] in bleeding patients. Lane et al.[82] and Ljungberg et al.[83] have compared low molecular weight heparinoids with conventional heparin as the sole dialysis anti-coagulant and demonstrated adequate suppression of fibrin formation (as judged by fibrinopeptide A levels) coupled with prolonged WBACT. In both cases, a single intravenous bolus of approximately 5000 anti-factor Xa units was adequate to cover a 4 h haemodialysis. Lane et al.[82] also recommend a bolus of 4000 iu followed by 750 iu/h. Simple assays for anti-factor Xa activity are being developed and these

97

should provide better control during dialysis[84].

Despite these encouraging results, larger scale controlled trials will be required to assess the efficacy of these compounds in reducing bleeding risks while providing adequate dialysis anticoagulation. At the very least they may be useful in patients with heparin-induced thrombocytopenia or heparin allergies.

Epoprostenol (prostacyclin)

Epoprostenol is an endogenously produced prostanoid synthesized in vascular endothelium from platelet-derived endoperoxides by epoprostenol synthetase. Its main actions are to inhibit platelet aggregation and adhesion, thus helping to prevent thrombogenesis. Its action is mediated by adenylcyclase which leads to an increase in cyclic AMP in the platelets. Its action is opposed by thromboxane A_2 produced in the platelets from the same endoperoxide precursors as epoprostenol. At sites of vascular injury, thromboxane production predominates and platelet aggregation and activation occur. Epoprostenol inhibits platelet aggregation at much lower concentrations than are required to limit adhesion; this allows essential vascular repair to be initiated (i.e. platelet–collagen interaction) while platelet-rich thrombus formation is limited.

In haemodialysis membranes, a significant contribution to fibrin activation and thrombogenesis would be removed if the aggregation of platelets could be limited. These considerations led Woods et al.[85] successfully to use epoprostenol as the sole anticoagulant in haemodialysis in dogs.

Epoprostenol has been fairly extensively evaluated as an anticoagulant in haemodialysis. Turney et al.[86] reported a 'heparin-sparing' effect of epoprostenol while Zusman et al.[87] initiated studies using epoprostenol alone. They induced satisfactory anticoagulation with no evidence of activation of the intrinsic clotting system or fibrin formation. Eighty per cent of the patients studied had side effects, including hypotension, flushing and nausea, which disappeared shortly after cessation of the epoprostenol. Smith et al.[88] repeated this work, again noting side effects and some dialyser clotting, and, in addition, demonstrated an apparent increase in efficiency of haemodialysis in the patients treated with epoprostenol. Other investigators have since confirmed most of these findings[89-91]. Several reports suggest that there is a significant incidence of dialyser fibrin formation with epoprostenol as the sole anticoagulant and that increasing dosage to compensate for this leads to unacceptable side effects. Combination with low-dose heparin reduces these problems[92-94].

The optimal dosage for epoprostenol in haemodialysis (personal observation) would seem to be 5 ng/kg/min started shortly prior to haemodialysis. A bolus of heparin (1000 iu) should also be given and further doses of heparin judged on hourly assessment of whole blood activated clotting time, aiming to maintain this value at 120% of control.

Although the heparin-sparing effects of epoprostenol will guarantee its place in the management of high-bleeding-risk acute or chronic dialysis anticoagulation, its relatively high cost, instability once in solution and high incidence of side effects will limit its usefulness on a wide scale.

Chemically stable epoprostenol analogues are being developed and evaluated[95].

Citrate regional anticoagulation

Regional anticoagulation of the dialyser with heparin neutralized by protamine is difficult to control and may lead to bleeding complications. For at-risk patients, Pinnick et al.[96] and Hocken et al.[97] have suggested the use of citrate as the anticoagulant. Trisodium citrate dihydrate solution complexes ionized calcium, thus inducing anticoagulation. It is infused into the dialysis circuit before the dialyser; most of the citrate is removed by dialysis[98] and the remainder neutralized by transmembrane diffusion of calcium from dialysate[97]. Concomitant infusion of calcium chloride after the dialyser may help to neutralize remaining citrate[96]. Monitoring of the anticoagulant effect is by WBACT. Side effects are those of hypocalcaemia (tetany, paraesthesia, arrhythmias) and can be countered by administration of ionized calcium.

FUTURE DEVELOPMENTS

Major developments in dialysis anticoagulation will take two directions. Firstly, the development of new more-biocompatible membranes, possibly impregnated with anticoagulants, will limit the requirement for regional or systemic anticoagulation. Secondly, existing compounds and their use will be refined in the context of better understanding of the coagulation system. Low molecular weight heparinoids, which seem to separate the anticoagulant from the haemorrhagic and platelet aggregating effects of heparin, are particularly interesting.

Finally, the original dialysis anticoagulant, hirudin, is now available in recombinant form. It has a specific reaction with thrombin, does not require a plasma cofactor and has no effect on platelets[99]. After seventy-five years of development, anticoagulation for haemodialysis has come full circle!

REFERENCES

1. Abel, J. J., Rowntree, L. G. and Turner, B. B. (1913). On the removal of diffusible substances from the circulating blood by means of dialysis. *Trans. Assoc. Am. Physicians*, **28**, 51
2. Abel, J. J., Rowntree, L. G. and Turner, B. B. (1913). On the removal of diffusible substances from the circulating blood of living animals by dialysis. *J. Pharmacol. Exp. Ther.*, **5**, 275
3. Drukker, W. (1983). Haemodialysis – a historical review. In Drukker, W. (ed.) *Replacement of Renal Function by Dialysis*, pp. 3–52. (Boston: Martinus Nijhoff)
4. Thalhimer, W. (1937). Experimental exchange transfusion for reducing azotaemia. *Proc. Soc. Exp. Biol. Med.*, **37**, 641
5. Blakely, J. A. (1968). A rapid bedside method for the control of heparin therapy. *Can. Med. Assoc. J.*, **99**, 1072
6. Shanklin, N. and Ploth, D. W. (1980). Evaluation of an activated clotting time technique for use in haemodialysis. *Dial. Transplant.*, **9**, 995
7. Estes, J. W. (1970). Kinetics of the anticoagulant effect of heparin. *J. Am. Med. Assoc.*, **212**, 1492–1495
8. Congdon, J. E., Kardinal, C. G. and Wallin, J. D. (1973). Monitoring heparin therapy in haemodialysis. *J. Am. Med. Assoc.*, **226**, 1529
9. Lindsay, R. M. (1983). Practical use of anticoagulants. In Drukker, W. (ed.) *Replacement of Renal Function by Dialysis*, pp. 201–222. (Boston, Martinus Nijhoff)
10. Saniabadi, A. R., Lowe, G. D. O., Forbes, C. D., Prentice, C. R. M. and Barbenel, J. C. (1984). The role of red blood cells in spontaneous aggregation of platelets

in whole blood. In Paul, J. P. and Gaylor, J. D. S. (eds.) *Biomaterials in Artificial Organs*, pp. 249–257. (London: MacMillan)
11. Riesman, D. (1907). Hemorrhages in the course of Bright's Disease with a nephrotic origin. *Am. J. Med. Sci.*, **134**, 709
12. Rabiner, S. F. (1972). Uremic bleeding. *Prog. Haemostasis Thromb.*, **1**, 233
13. Castaldi, P. A., Rosenberg, M. C. and Stewart, J. H. (1966). The bleeding disorder of uraemia. *Lancet*, **2**, 66–69
14. Donner, L. (1960). The hemostatic defect of acute and chronic uraemia. *Thromb. Diath. Haemorrh.*, **5**, 319
15. Salzman, E. W. and Neri, L. L. (1966). Adhesiveness of blood platelets in uremia. *Thromb. Diath. Haemorrh.*, **15**, 84
16. Steward, J. H. and Castaldi, P. A. (1967). Uraemic bleeding – A reversible platelet defect corrected by dialysis. *Q. J. Med.*, **36**, 409–423
17. Rabiner, S. F and Hrodek, O. (1968). Platelet factor 3 in normal subjects and patients with renal failure. *J. Clin. Invest.*, **47**, 901
18. Lindsay, R. M., Moorthy, A. V., Koens, F. and Linton, A. L. (1975). Platelet function in dialysed and non-dialysed patients with chronic renal failure. *Clin. Nephrol.*, **4**, 52–57
19. Lindsay, R. M., Friesen, M., Aronstam, A., Andrus, F., Clark, W. F. and Linton, A. L. (1978). Improvement of platelet function by increased frequency of haemodialysis. *Clin. Nephrol.*, **10**, 67–70
20. Gallice, P., Fournier, N., Crevat, A., Saingra, S., Frayssinet, R., Murisasco, A. and Sicardi, F. (1980). 'In vitro' inhibition of platelet aggregation by uremic middle molecules. *Biomedicine*, **33**, 185–188
21. Kazatchkine, M., Sultan, Y., Caen, J. P. and Bariety, J. (1976). Bleeding in renal failure – a possible cause. *Br. Med. J.*, **2**, 612–614
22. Vaziri, N. D., Toohey, J., Paule, S., Alikhani, S. and Hung, E. (1984). Coagulation abnormalities in patients with end stage renal failure treated with haemodialysis. *Int. J. Artif. Organs*, **7**, 323–326
23. Lindsay, R. M., Prentice, C. R. M., Davidson, J. F., Burton, J. A. and McNicol, G. P. (1972). Haemostatic changes during dialysis associated with thrombus formation on dialysis membrane. *Br. Med. J.*, **4**, 454–458
24. Harter, J. R., Burch, J. W., Majerus, P. W., Stanford, N., Delmez, J. A., Anderson, C. B. and Weerts, C. A. (1979). *N. Engl. J. Med.*, **301**, 577–579
25. Kaegi, A., Pines, G. F., Shimizu, A., Trivedi, H., Hirsh, J. and Geat, M. (1974). Arterio-venous shunt thrombosis: prevention by sulphinpyrazone. *N. Engl. J. Med.*, **290**, 304–306
26. Bischel, M. D., Scoles, B. G. and Mohler, J. G. (1975). Evidence for pulmonary microembolization during hemodialysis. *Chest*, **67**, 335–337
27. Turney, J. H., Williams, L. C., Fewell, M. R., Parsons, V. and Weston, M. J. (1980). Platelet protection and heparin sparing with prostacyclin during regular dialysis therapy. *Lancet*, **2**, 219–222
28. George, C. P. R., Slichter, S. J., Quadracci, L. J., Striker, G. E. and Harker, L. A. (1974). A kinetic evaluation of hemostasis in renal disease. *N. Engl. J. Med.*, **293**, 1111–1115
29. Smith, D., Santhanam, S. and Krumlovsky, F. A. (1979). Beta-thromboglobulin in patients with chronic renal failure – effect of haemodialysis. *Clin. Res.*, **27**, 296
30. Smith, M. C. and Dunn, M. J. (1981). Impaired platelet thromboxane production in renal failure. *Nephron*, **29**, 133–137

31. Jorgenson, K. A. and Ingeborg, S. (1979). Platelets and platelet function in patients with chronic uraemia on maintenance haemodialysis. *Nephron*, **23**, 233–236
32. Bemis, J., Rigney, J., Sosin, A. and Deane, N. (1977). Enhanced platelet aggregation in chronic renal failure patients receiving haemodialysis treatment. *Trans. Am. Soc. Artif. Intern. Organs*, **23**, 48–52
33. Viener, A., Aviram, M., Betler, O. S. and Brook, J. G. (1986). Enhanced in vitro platelet aggregation in haemodialysis patients. *Nephron*, **43**, 139–143
34. Charvat, J., König, J. and Bláha, J. (1986). Is heparin responsible for enhanced platelet aggregation after haemodialysis? *Nephron*, **44**, 89–91
35. Nenci, G. G., Berretini, M., Angelli, G., Parise, P., Buoneristiani, V. and Ballatori, E. (1979). Effects of peritoneal dialysis, haemodialysis and kidney transplantation on blood platelet function. *Nephron*, **23**, 287–292
36. Schondorf, T. H. and Hey, D. (1974). Platelet function tests in uraemia and under acetylsalicylic acid administration. *Haemostasis*, **3**, 129–136
37. Zucker, M. B. (1977). Biological effects of heparin action. Heparin and platelet function. *Fed. Proc.*, **36**, 47–49
38. Brash, J. L. and Lyman, D. J. (1971). Adsorption of proteins and lipids to nonbiological surfaces. In Hair, M. L. (ed.) *The Chemistry of Biosurfaces*, p. 177. (New York: Marcel Dekker)
39. Hakim, R. M. (1986). Clinical sequelae of complement activation in haemodialysis. *Clin. Nephrol.*, **26**, S9–S12
40. Gunnarsson, B., Asaba, H., Kiibus, A., Soderborg, B., Wiklund, S. and Bergstrom, J. (1979). Fibrin deposition in disposable dialysers before and after reuse. *Clin. Nephrol.*, **12**, 117–121
41. Niemetz, J., Muhlfelder, T., Chierego, M. E. and Troy, B. (1977). Procoagulant activity of leucocytes. *Ann. N.Y. Acad. Sci.*, **283**, 208–211
42. Hakim, R. A. (1985). Biocompatibility issues in haemodialysis. *Proc. Eur. Dial. Transpl. Assoc.*, **22**, 163–170
43. Agresti, J., Conroy, J. D., Olshan, A., Conney, J. F., Schwartz, A., Brodsky, I., Krevlin, L. and Chinitz, J. (1985). Heparin-free haemodialysis with cuprophane hollow fibre dialysers by a frequent saline flush, high blood flow technique. *Trans. Am. Soc. Artif. Intern. Organs*, **21**, 590–593
44. Casati, S., Moia, M., Graziani, G., Cantaluppi, A., Citterio, A., Mannucci, P. M. and Ponticelli, C. (1984). Haemodialysis without anticoagulants: efficiency and haemostatic aspects. *Clin. Nephrol.*, **21**, 102–105
45. Stiekema, J. C. J. (1986). Heparin and its biocompatibility. *Clin. Nephrol.*, **26**, S3–S8
46. Tollefsen, D. M., Magerus, D. W. and Blank, M. W. (1984). Heparin cofactor II. Purification and properties of a heparin dependent inhibitor of thrombin in human plasma. *J. Biol. Chem.*, **257**, 2162–2168
47. Williman, P., Alig, A. and Binswanger, U. (1979). Minimal intermittent heparinisation during haemodialysis. *Nephron*, **23**, 191–193
48. Biggs, R. (1972). *Human Blood Coagulation, Haemostasis and Thrombosis.* (London: Blackwell)
49. Salzman, E. W., Deykin, D. and Shapiro, R. M. (1980). Effect of heparin and heparin fractions on platelet aggregation. *J. Clin. Invest.*, **65**, 64
50. Lins, L. E., Ljungberg, B. and Söderström, P. O. (1987). Heparin requirement in haemodialysis, a comparison between single needle and two needle dialysis. *Clin. Nephrol.*, **28**, 102–103

51. Mingardi, G., Perico, N., Pusineri, F., Massazza, M., Marchesi, E., Mecca, G., Remuzzi, G. and Donati, M. B. (1984). Heparin for haemodialysis: Practical guidelines for administration and monitoring. *Int. J. Artif. Organs*, **7**, 269–274

52. Wilhelmsson, S., Asaba, H., Gunnarsson, B., Kudryk, B., Robinson, D. and Bergström, J. (1981). Measurement of fibrinopeptide A in the evaluation of heparin activity and fibrin formation during haemodialysis. *Clin. Nephrol.*, **15**, 252–258

53. Wollin, A. and Jaques, L. B. (1972). Analysis of heparin – Azure A metachromasy in agarose gel. *Can. J. Physiol. Pharmacol.*, **50**, 65–71

54. Ross, R. L., Whittlesey, F. H., Splittgerber, F. H., Salley, S. O. and Klein, M. D. (1986). Rapid assay for heparin during extracorporeal circulation. *Trans. Am. Soc. Artif. Intern. Organs*, **32**, 274–277

55. Gotch, F. A. and Keen, M. L. (1977). Precise control of minimal heparinisation for high bleeding risk haemodialysis. *Trans. Am. Soc. Artif. Intern. Organs*, **23**, 168–176

56. Farell, P. C., Ward, R., Schindhelm, K. and Gotch, F. A. (1978). Precise anticoagulation for routine haemodialysis. *J. Lab. Clin. Med.*, **92**, 164–176

57. Khazine, F. and Simons, O. (1985). Pharmacokinetic monitoring of heparin therapy for regular haemodialysis. *Artif. Organs*, **9**, 59–61

58. Swartz, R. D. (1981). Haemorrhage during high risk hemodialysis using controlled heparin. *Nephron*, **28**, 65–69

59. Maher, J. F, Lapierre, L., Schreiner, G. E., Geiger, M. and Westervelt, F. B. (1963). Regional heparinisation for haemodialysis. *N. Engl. J. Med.*, **268**, 451–456

60. Lindholm, D. D. and Murray, J. S. (1964). A simplified method of regional herpainisation during haemodialysis according to a predetermined dosage formula. *Trans. Am. Soc. Artif. Intern. Organs*, **10**, 92–97

61. Swartz, R. D. and Port, F. K. (1979). Preventing haemorrhage in high risk haemodialysis: Regional versus low-dose heparin. *Kidney Int.*, **16**, 513–518

62. Kaplan, A. A. and Pettrillo, R. (1987). Regional heparinisation for continuous arterio-venous hemofiltration (CAVH). *Trans. Am. Soc. Artif. Intern. Organs*, **33**, 312–315

63. Janson, P. A., Moake, J. L. and Carpinito, G. (1983). Aspirin prevents heparin-induced platelet aggregation in vivo. *Br. J. Haematol.*, **53**, 166–168

64. Miller, L. C., Hall, J. C. and Crow, J. W. (1985). Haemodialysis in heparin-associated thrombocytopenia: Epoprostenol (PGI$_2$) as sole anticoagulant. *Dial. Transplant*, **14**, 579–580

65. Leehey, D. J., Kanak, R. J., Messmore, H. L., Nawab, Z. M., Popli, S. and Ing, T. S. (1987). Heparin-associated thrombocytopenia in maintenance haemodialysis patients. *Int. J. Artif. Intern. Organs*, **10**, 390–392

66. Cines, D. B., Kaywin, P., Bina, M., Tomaski, A. and Schreiber, A. D. (1980). Heparin-associated thrombocytopenia. *N. Engl. J. Med.*, **303**, 788–795

67. King, D. J. and Kelton, J. G. (1984). Heparin-associated thrombocytopenia. *Ann. Int. Med.*, **100**, 535–540

68. Bell, W. R. and Royall, R. M. (1980). Heparin-associated thrombocytopenia: A comparison of three heparin preparations. *N. Engl. J. Med.*, **303**, 902–907

69. Chang, B. H., Pitney, W. R. and Castaldi, P. A. (1982). Heparin-induced thrombocytopenia: Association of thrombotic complications with heparin-dependent

IgG antibody that induces thromboxane synthesis and platelet aggregation. *Lancet*, **2**, 1246–1248

70. Brace, L. D. and Fareed, I. (1985). An objective assessment of the interaction of heparin and its fragments with human platelets. *Semin. Thromb. Haemostasis*, **11**, 190–196

71. Brandt, P., Jespersen, J. and Sorensen, L. H. (1981). Antithrombin-III and platelets in haemodialysis patients. *Nephron*, **28**, 1–3

72. Turney, J. H., Fewell, L. C., Williams, M. D. and Weston, M. J. (1982). Paradoxical behaviour of antithrombin-III during haemodialysis and its prevention with prostacyclin. *Clin. Nephrol.*, **17**, 31–35

73. Leonard, A. and Shapiro, F. L. (1975). Subdural haematoma in regularly haemodialysed patients. *Ann. Int. Med.*, **82**, 650–652

74. Silverberg, S., Oreopoulos, D. G. and Wise, D. J. (1977). Pericarditis in patients undergoing long-term haemodialysis and peritoneal dialysis. *Am. J. Med.*, **63**, 874–876

75. Milutinovich, J., Folette, W. C. and Schribner, B. H. (1977). Spontaneous retroperitoneal bleeding in patients on chronic haemodialysis. *Ann. Int. Med.*, **86**, 189

76. Galen, M. A., Steinberg, S. M. and Lowrie, E. G. (1975). Haemorrhagic pleural effusion in patients undergoing chronic haemodialysis. *Ann. Int. Med.*, **82**, 359–362

77. Korz, R. (1971). Heparin-induzierte mobilisation von calcium und anorgischem phosphat in zusammenhang mit extraössaren verkalkungen bei chronisher hämodialyse. *Klin. Wschr.*, **49**, 684–688

78. Bergrem, H. and Leivestad, T. (1978). Dialysis death and increased free fatty acids. *Lancet*, **2**, 1160

79. Holmer, E., Lindahl, U., Backstrom, G., Thunberg, L., Soderstrom, G. and Andersson, L. O. (1980). Anticoagulant activities and effects on platelets of a heparin fragment with a high affinity for anti-thrombin. *Thromb. Res.*, **18**, 861–865

80. Salzman, E. W., Deykin, D. and Shapiro, R. M. (1980). Effect of heparin and heparin fractions on platelet aggregation. *J. Clin. Invest.*, **65**, 64–66

81. Henny, Ch.P., Ten Cate, H. and Ten Cate, J. W. (1983). Use of a new heparinoid as anticoagulant during acute haemodialysis of patients with bleeding complications. *Lancet*, **1**, 890–891

82. Lane, D. A., Ireland, H., Flynn, A., Anastassiades, E. and Curtis, J. R. (1986). Haemodialysis with low MW Heparin: Dosage requirements for the elimination of extracorporeal fibrin formation. *Nephrol. Dial. Transplant.*, **1**, 179–187

83. Ljungberg, B., Blomback, M., Johnsson, H. and Lins, L. E. (1987). A single dose of a low molecular weight heparin fragment for anticoagulation during haemodialysis. *Clin. Nephrol.*, **27**, 31–35

84. Handeland, G. (1986). Simplified chromogenic substrate assay for low molecular weight heparin. *Thromb. Res.*, **42**, 105–108

85. Woods, H. F., Ash, G. and Weston, M. J. (1978). Prostacyclin can replace herapin in haemodialysis in dogs. *Lancet*, **2**, 1075–1077

86. Turney, J. H., Williams, L. C., Fewell, M. R., Parsons, V. and Weston, M. J. (1980). Platelet protection and heparin sparing with prostacyclin during regular dialysis therapy. *Lancet*, **2**, 219–222

87. Zusman, R. M., Rubin, R. H., Cato, A. E., Cocchetto, D. M., Crow, J. W. and Tolkoff-Rubin, N. (1981). Haemodialysis using prostacyclin instead of heparin

as the sole antithrombotic agent. *N. Engl. J. Med.*, **304**, 934–939
88. Smith, M. C, Danviriyasup, K., Crow, J. W., Cato, A. E., Park, G. D., Hassid, A. and Dunn, M. J. (1982). Prostacyclin substitution for heparin in long-term hemodialysis. *Am. J. Med.*, **73**, 669–677
89. Turney, J. H., Dodd, N. J. and Weston, M. J. (1981). Prostacyclin in extra-corporeal circulations. *Lancet*, **1**, 1101
90. Arze, R. S. and Ward, M. K. (1981). Prostacyclin safer than heparin in haemo-dialysis. *Lancet*, **2**, 50
91. Rylance, P. B. (1984). Haemodialysis with prostacyclin (epoprostenol) alone. *Proc. Eur. Dial. Transplant. Assoc.*, **21**, 281–286
92. Knudsen, F., Nielsen, A. H., Kornerup, H. J., Pedersen, J. C. and Dyerberg, J. (1984). Epoprostenol as sole antithrombotic treatment during haemodialysis. *Lancet*, **2**, 235–236
93. Keogh, A. M., Rylance, P. B., Weston, M. J. and Parsons, V. (1984). Prostacyclin (epoprostenol) haemodialysis in patients at risk of haemorrhage. *Proc. Eur. Dial. Transplant. Nurs. Assoc.*, **13**, 51–53
94. Rylance, P. B., Gordge, M. P., Keogh, A. M., Parsons, V. and Weston, M. J. (1984) Epoprostenol during haemodialysis. *Lancet*, **2**, 744–745
95. Suzuki, T., Naganuma, S., Takahashi, K. and Ota, K. (1986). Carbacyclin derivative (CS-570) – a new anticoagulant for haemodialysis. *Trans. Am. Soc. Artif. Intern. Organs*, **32**, 291–296
96. Pinnick, R. V., Weighmann, T. B. and Diedrich, D. A. (1983). Regional citrate anticoagulation for haemodialysis in the patient at high risk for bleeding. *N. Engl. J. Med.*, **308**, 258–261
97. Hocken, A. G. and Hurst, P. L. (1987). Citrate regional anticoagulation in haemo-dialysis. *Nephron*, **46**, 7–10
98. Winchester, J. F., Gelfand, M. C., Knepshield, J. H. and Schreiner, G. E. (1977). Dialysis and haemoperfusion of drugs – update. *Trans. Am. Soc. Artif. Intern. Organs*, **23**, 762–842
99. Markwardt, F., Nowak, G., Stürzebecker, J., Griessbach, U., Walsmann, P. and Vogel, G. (1984). Pharmacokinetics and anticoagulant effect of hirudin in man. *Thromb. Haemostasis*, **52**, 160–163

INDEX

acetaldehyde, arterial levels,
 acetate/bicarbonate
 dialysis 12–13
acetate
 arterial pressure effects 14–16
 dialysis buffer 3
 kinetic modelling studies 12
 metabolism, Krebs cycle 2–3, 18
 myocardial contractility effects 13–16
acetate dialysis
 base repletion 20
 net mass transfer, acetate
  intolerance 8–9
 plasma levels 5–6, 11–13
 pyruvate levels 19
 utilization rate 3
acetate intolerance 4, 5–12
 acetate net mass transfer 8–9
 blood acetate levels 11–13
 CRT scores 9, 10
 dialysate sodium concentration 8, 9–10
 elderly patients 8
acetoacetate, levels, acetate dialysis 19, 20
acetoacetyl CoA, ketone
  body/cholesterol synthesis 2, 6
n-acetylcysteine, drug chelation 70, 71
acid-base balance
 acetate/bicarbonate dialysis 19–21
 haemofiltration 46

ADP, release, basic platelet reaction 87
adriamycin, removal 74
adult respiratory distress syndrome
  (ARDS), haemofiltration 46–7
aluminium osteomalacia 52
aluminium overload 71
alveolar–arterial oxygen gradient,
  dialusis 17
alveolar ventilation, acetate dialysis
  18
amitriptyline poisoning 70
analgesics, removal,
  haemoperfusion 67
anticancer agents, removal,
  haemoperfusion 67, 74
anticoagulation
 dialysis 92–3
 rebound, post-dialysis 96
 regional 99
antidepressants, removal,
  haemoperfusion 67
antimicrobials, removal,
  haemoperfusion 67
antiplasmins 84
antirheumatic agents, removal,
  haemoperfusion 67
antithrombin III 84, 86
apoprotein C II deficiency 22
arachidonate, cyclo-oxygenase
  pathway 88
arterial oxygen tension (PaO_2),
  reduction, causes 17

asymmetric polymers, haemofiltration
    membranes 37–8
ATP
    bicarbonate regeneration 2, 4
    release, basic platelet reaction 87
autonomic neuropathy
    acetate/bicarbonate dialysate 8
    low sodium/bicarbonate dialysate 8,
        9–10, 11

barbiturates, removal,
        haemoperfusion 67, 69
basic platelet reaction 87–8
bicarbonate
    arterial pressure effects 14–16
    plasma levels
        acetate dialysis 6
        haemofiltration 46
    regeneration 2, 4, 19, 20
bicarbonate dialysis
    acetate plasma levels 12
    buffer repletion 21
    cost effectiveness 24, 25
    geographical aspects 24–5
    patient choice guidelines 24–5
    patients treated 23
biliary peritonitis, ARDS 47
bilirubin removal, haemoperfusion 75
bleeding time 91
blood flow rates, haemofiltration 35–6,
        37
Bohr effect 17
bovine grafts, haemofiltration in
        children 53
breast cancer, staphylococcal A protein,
        haemoperfusion 75
bronchopneumonia, ARDS 47

C1 inhibitor 84
calcium
    balance, haemofiltration 51–2
    solubility, bicarbonate dialysate 2
CAPD
    diabetes mellitus 54, 55
    survival rates 54
carbon dioxide tension, acetate
        dialysis 18
carbon haemoperfusion, uraemia 64

cardiodepression, acetate-
        associated 13–16
cardiovascular drugs, removal,
        haemoperfusion 67
cardiovascular stability
    acetate/bicarbonate dialysis 13–16
    haemofiltration 45–6
    HF/dialysis 50
carpal tunnel syndrome, HF/dialysis
        association 53
CAVH 42
    acute renal failure 43–4
    HF/dialysis differences 44–8, 49
    heparinization bleeding 44
    indications 43
    infants 53
    problems/risks 43–4
    regional heparinization 96
cerebral oedema, hepatic coma 72
charcoal haemoperfusion
    drug removal 68, 69
    fulminant hepatic
        encephalopathy 72, 73
    uraemia 64–7
chelators, drug poisoning 70, 71
children, haemofiltration 53
choice reaction time, acetate level
        effects 9, 10
Cimino fistulae, haemofiltration in
        children 53
citrate
    acetate dialysis 18, 19
    metabolism, oxygen
        consumption 18
    regional anticoagulation 99
coagulation
    abnormalities, hepatic failure 72
    assessment, dialysis 89–91
    cascades, intrinsic/extrinsic 85–6
    system 84
    see also anticoagulation
coagulation factors
    activation 85–6
    haemoperfusion effects 63
coma, hepatic 72–4
complement
    activation, membrane-induced 17
    components, platelet
        aggregation 92–3

continuous arteriovenous
    haemofiltration *see* CAVH
creatinine removal
    haemofiltration/dialysis 47, 48, 52
    haemoperfusion 66

dementia, dialysis 71
diabetes mellitus,
    haemofiltration/CAPD 54–5
dialyser surface area,
    acetate/bicarbonate net mass
    transfer 8–9
digitalis poisoning 69, 70, 75
digoxin
    poisoning, immunoadsorption 75
    removal 69
disseminated intravascular coagulation,
    renal failure 92
DNA-collodion coated charcoal,
    haemoperfusion, SLE 75
drug intoxication,
    haemoperfusion/dialysis 67, 68–
    71
dysrhythmias, acute renal/respiratory
    failure 45

EEG, acetate/bicarbonate dialysate
    effects 9
elderly
    acetate intolerance 8
    haemofiltration, survival rates 54
    treatment-associated disorders 48
electromyogram, uraemia,
    haemoperfusion effects 66
encephalopathy 71
    see also hepatic encephalopathy
epoprostenol (prostacyclin) 61, 64, 98–
    9
    heparin combination 99
    synthesis 88
ethanol poisoning 70
ethylene glycol poisoning 70

factor VIII–von Willebrand
    activity 86, 92
fat-soluble drugs, removal,
    haemoperfusion 68
fatty acids, synthesis, malonyl CoA 2,
    5

febrile reactions, haemofiltration 54–5
fibrin, degradation products 90
fibrinogen
    assay 90
    degradation products (FDP) 90
    plasma levels, haemoperfusion 63
fibrinolytic system 84, 86–7
fibrinopeptide A 90
fibronectin, plasma levels,
    haemoperfusion 63

Gambro haemofiltration system 38
gases, removal, haemoperfusion 67
gluconeogenesis 19–20
glutethimide, removal 69
glycogenolysis 19–20
growth hormone 52

haemodialysis (HD)
    biochemical changes 47, 48
    CAVH/haemofiltration
        differences 44–8, 49
    guidelines 69, 71
    haemofiltration clearance
        comparisons 34
    haemoperfusion combination,
        uraemia 66
    historical aspects 1–2
    patients treated 23
    survival rates 54
haemofiltration (HF)
    acute renal failure 43–8
    biochemical changes 47, 48
    CAVH/haemodialysis
        differences 44–8, 49
    children 53
    chronic renal failure 48–56
    definition 33
    dialysis clearance comparisons 34
    dialysis differences 33–4
    equipment 38–42
    filter specifications 38
    indications 56
    long-term results 53–5
    materials 37–8, 39
    metabolic effects 52–3
    monitor 38–9, 40, 41
        functions 39–40
    patients treated 23

haemofiltration (HF) – *contd*
  performance variables 35–7
  postdilution 34, 35
  predilution 34–5
  principles 33–5
  quantitation 56
  side effects 63–4, 66
  staff training 43
  Starling effect 15
  survival rates 54
  systems available 38, 41–2
haemoglobin, oxygen affinity, blood pH
    17
haemoperfusion (HP)
  costs 66
  devices available 62
  haemodialysis combination,
      uraemia 66
  principles 61–3
  sorbents 61–2
haemostatic system 84–91
HDL
  Apo-A1 levels, bicarbonate
      dialysis 22
  cholesterol fraction 22
  triglyceride fraction levels,
      bicarbonate dialysis 22
heparin 61
  administration regimens 94–6
  adverse effects 96–7
  bleeding complications 96
  chemical assay 95
  clotting factor inactivation 94
  haemodialysis use 94–6
  platelet interaction 94
  structure/actions 93–4
heparinization
  control 95
  regional 95–6
heparinoids, low molecular weight 97–
    8
hepatic coma, haemoperfusion,
      prostacyclin 64
hepatic encephalopathy
  hemoperfusion 72–4
  pathogenesis 72
hepatic failure, haemoperfusion 72–4
haepatorenal failure, dialysis acetate
      levels 12

herbicides, removal,
      haemoperfusion 67
high molecular weight molecules,
      removal, HF/dialysis 52
hirudin 100
hydrophilic gel polymers,
      haemofiltration
      membranes 37–8
β-hydroxybutyrate, levels, acetate
      dialysis 19, 20
hypercatabolism, haemofiltration 47
hyperlipoproteinaemia 22–3
hypertension
  control, haemofiltration 50, 51
  volume-dependent 51
  volume-independent 51
hypertriglyceridaemia
  acetate/bicarbonate dialysis 22–3
  VLDL levels 22
hypnotics, removal,
      haemoperfusion 67
hypotension
  acetate/bicarbonate dialysis, elderly
      patients 8
  HF/dialysis association 48–50
  ultrafiltration-induced 45
hypothyroidism, T4/TBG ratio 52
hypoxaemia, dialysis association 17–18
hypoxia, acetate/bicarbonate
      dialysis 18

immune protein, adsorption,
      haemoperfusion 75
insecticides, removal,
      haemoperfusion 67
interleukin 1, PGE_2-induced
      vasodilation 46
intermediary metabolism,
      acetate/bicarbonate dialysis 19–
      21
ion-exchange resin haemoperfusion 64
  drug removal 68, 69
iron overload 71

kallikrein, factor XII activation 85
ketogenesis 20
kininogen, high molecular weight, factor
      XII activation 85
Kolff's dialysate formulation 2

LDL-ApoB levels, bicarbonate
    dialysis 22
leukocytes, dialyser membrane, platelet
    aggregation 92–3
leukopenia, haemoperfusion-
    associated 63
lipid metabolism, heparin effects 97
lipid-soluble drugs, removal,
    haemoperfusion 68
lipids, removal 75
lipoprotein lipase (LPL), deficiency 22
low molecular weight heparinoids 97–8

magnesium, solubility, bicarbonate
    dialysate 2
malignant disease, haemofiltration 54
membranes
    biocompatible 92–3, 95, 100
    coagulation effects 92–3
    complement activation 17
    haemofiltration 37–8, 39
    leukocyte, platelet aggregation 92–3
metabolic acidosis, acetate/bicarbonate
    dialysis 19–21
metabolic alkalosis, oxygen
    transport/ventilation (Bohr) 17
methanol poisoning 70
methotrexate, removal 74
β_2-microglobulin, removal,
    haemofiltration 53
muscle cramps, HF/dialysis
    association 48–50
myocardial contractility, acetate
    effects 13–16
myocardinal infarction,
    haemofiltration 54

nausea/vomiting, HF/dialysis
    association 48–50
nerve conduction velocity, uraemic,
    haemoperfusion effects 66
neuropathy, diabetic,
    haemofiltration/CAPD 55
neutropenia, transient, dialysis 17
nortriptyline poisoning 70

oliguria, diuretic-unresponsive 43
organic ion production,
    acetate/bicarbonate dialysis 20

osteitis fibrosa 52
osteodystrophy, reneal 51–2, 71
osteomalacia 71
    aluminium associated 52
oxygen tension, dialysis 17

paracetamol poisoning 69
    n-acetylcysteine 70
paraquat poisoning 69, 70
parathyroid hormone, levels,
    haemofiltration 51–2
partial thromboplastin time (PTT) 90,
    95
pericarditis, uraemic, haemoperfusion
    effects 66
peritoneal dialysis, survival rates 54
phosphate removal, haemofiltration 51
phospholipids, platelet membrane 84,
    86
plasmin 84, 87
    activity assessment 90
plasminogen, activation 87
platelet adherence 84
platelet aggregation 84
    assessment 91
    complement components 92–3
    dialyser membrane leukocytes 92–3
    prostacyclin (epoprostenol)
        effects 98
platelet factor IV, release 87, 91
platelet function 87–9
    assessment 91
platelets
    activators 86, 87
    ADP/collagen activation 86
    basic reaction 87–8
    count, whole blood 91
    hyperactivity, dialysis 92
    membrane phospholipids,
        thromboxane A_2 84
    surface interaction 87–9
poisoning
    haemoperfusion/dialysis 67, 68–71
    metabolic abnormalities,
        haemodialysis 70
prostacyclin (epoprostenol) 61, 64, 98–
    9
    heparin combination 99
    synthesis 88

prostaglandin E_2, vasodilation
    induction, interleukin I   46
protein-bound drugs, removal,
    haemoperfusion   68
protein C   81, 84
proteins
    plasma, haemofiltration effects   35,
        36, 50-1
    platelet-specific, assessment   91
prothrombin time (PT)   90
pruritus, uraemic, haemoperfusion
    effects   66
psoriasis   74
pulmonary performance, dialysis
    effects   17-18
pyruvate, oxaloacetate synthesis   19

radial Scribner shunt,
    haemofiltration   44, 47, 53
red cells, secondary membrane
    shearing   35
regional heparinization, CAVH   96
renal failure
    acute
        cardiovascular stability   16
        CAVH   43-4
        haemofiltration   43-8
    cardiovascular events   45
    chronic, haemofiltration   48-56
    disseminated intravascular
        coagulation   92
renal osteodystrophy   51-2, 71
renal/respiratory failure,
    haemofiltration   46-7
reptilase coagulation test   90
resin haemoperfusion, hepatic coma   74
    see also ion-exchange resin; XAD-4
respiratory quotient, acetate
    metabolism   18
retinopathy, diabetic,
    haemofiltration/CAPD   55

salicylate poisoning   69, 70
schizophrenia, dialysis   74
sedatives, removal, haemoperfusion   67
serotonin, release, basic platelet
    reaction   87
SLE, DNA-collodion coated charcoal
    haemoperfusion   75

sodium, dialysate levels
    blood pressure effects   15, 16
    intradialytic symptom effects   8, 9-
        10, 11
solute clearance calculation,
    haemofiltration   36
solvent-drag, haemofiltration   33
solvents, removal, haemoperfusion   67
staphylococcal A protein, breast
    cancer   75
Starling effect, ultrafiltration-
    associated   15
subclavian cannulation,
    haemofiltration   44, 53

theophylline poisoning   69, 70-1
thrombi formation   84
thrombin time (TT)   90
thrombocytopenia, heparin-
    associated   96
β-thromboglobulin, release   87, 91
thrombotic/thromboembolic events
    dialysis   92, 96
    heparin-associated   96
thromboxane A_2
    platelet membrane phospholipids   84
    synthesis   88
thyroid stimulating hormone   52
thyroxine   52
tranquillizers, removal,
    haemoperfusion   67
transmembrane pressure,
    haemofiltration   35
treatment complications,
    haemofiltration   55-6
treatment-associated disorders
    elderly   48
    HF/dialysis comparisons   48-53
tri-iodothyronine   52

ultrafiltration rate, blood flow rate
    relationship   35-6
uraemia
    activated charcoal
        haemoperfusion   62
    bleeding tendency   92
    CAVH   43
    dialysis, thrombotic/thromboembolic
        events   92

haemoperfusion   63, 64–7
  haemodialysis combinations   66
solute adsorption,
  haemoperfusion   63–3
urea removal
  haemofiltration/dialysis   47, 48, 52
  haemoperfusion   66

vascular access, haemofiltration   44, 53, 54, 56
vasodilation, PGE$_2$-induced   46
ventricular arrhythmias, HF/dialysis
  association   50
ventricular function, dialysis effects   15, 16

VLDL
  impaired clearance   22
  serum levels,
    hypertriglyceridaemia   22

whole blood
  activated clotting time
    (WBACT)   89, 95
  activated partial thromboplastin time
    (WBAPTT)   90, 95
  clotting time (WBCT)   89, 95
  platelet count   91

XAD-4 resin haemoperfusion, drug
  removal   68, 69